PROACTIVE STEPS TO PREVENTING CANCER

Empowering Your Health Implement actionable steps focusing on diet, physical activity, and mental wellness and evidence-based practices for a healthier life

AXTON MARLOWE

Table of Contents

INTRODUCTION

Around the world, almost every person & family is affected by cancer. Cancer has a significant & wide-ranging effect, whether it is experienced personally or through a loved one's experience. There is hope, though, despite the fact that this illness is frequently debilitating. Our daily decisions, which include those related to nutrition, exercise, mental health, & a dedication to leading a healthier lifestyle, have the potential to lower our risk of developing cancer. In "Proactive Steps to Preventing Cancer," we examine the research & data supporting these lifestyle choices & offer doable, realistic recommendations that anyone can incorporate into their daily routine to reduce their risk of developing cancer.

With an emphasis on empowerment, education, & long-term well-being, this book is meant to serve as your guide to a healthier, cancer-preventive lifestyle. You'll discover how your journey to prevent cancer can be greatly aided by making educated choices about your diet, physical activity, & emotional & mental well-being. There is no doubt that eating a well-balanced, nutrient-dense diet, exercising frequently, & taking care of your mental health can lower your risk of developing many types of cancer, boost your immune system, & enhance your general quality of life.

In the upcoming chapters, we will examine the most recent findings & tried-&-true methods for preventing cancer, offering a comprehensive framework that blends useful advice with scientific support. You'll learn how to make small but effective dietary adjustments, like increasing your intake of plant-based foods, cutting back on processed foods, & utilising antioxidants. You'll also learn about the significant effects of exercise on the body's capacity to fight off cancer as well as on controlling weight. Another important topic covered in this book is mental wellness; it has been demonstrated that stress reduction, mindfulness, & developing an optimistic outlook boost immunity & help fend off chronic illnesses like cancer.

However, preventing cancer is more than just avoiding the illness; it's about leading a vibrant, resilient life where your body & mind are in balance. Instead of being overwhelming, the proactive actions described in this book are meant to be manageable, long-lasting adjustments that you can incorporate into your everyday routine. Every chapter provides a road map for implementing realistic, long-lasting adjustments that can lower your risk of developing cancer while improving your general health & wellbeing.

It is impossible to overestimate the significance of preventing cancer proactively. Our future health is permanently impacted by the decisions we make today. We can reduce our risks & create the conditions for a full, healthy life by making well-informed decisions. A call to action, "Proactive Steps to Preventing Cancer" is more than just a book. Give yourself the information & resources you need to take charge of your health, adopt a cancer-prevention lifestyle, & make an investment in a long & healthy future. One step at a time, we can all work together to create a world in which cancer is preventable rather than inevitable.

Let's begin this journey together & take the first step toward a healthier, more empowered future.

CHAPTER 1: NUTRITION & CANCER PREVENTION

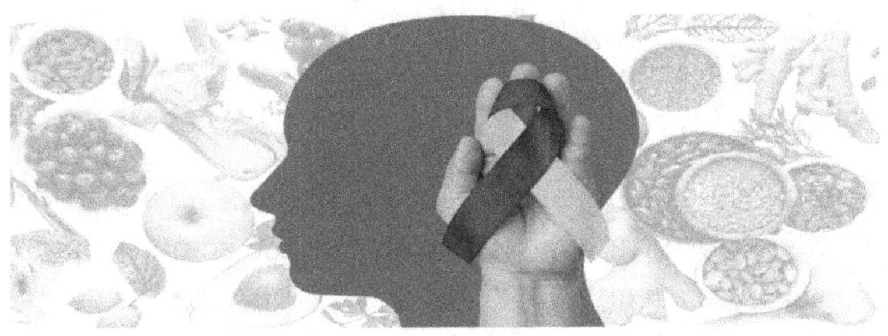

Scientific studies have repeatedly shown how important nutrition is in lowering the risk of cancer in recent decades. The intricate biological functions of our bodies, such as immune system function, DNA repair, & cell growth, are directly impacted by the food we consume. It has been demonstrated that eating a diet high in whole foods & low in processed foods, refined sugars, & unhealthy fats can dramatically reduce the risk of developing some types of cancer. On the other hand, diets heavy in trans fats, sugary drinks, & processed meats are linked to a higher risk of breast, colorectal, & other cancers. Examining not only specific foods but also more comprehensive dietary patterns & the complex interactions between macro- & micronutrients on cellular health is necessary to comprehend the relationship between nutrition & cancer. Because of their anti-inflammatory & antioxidant qualities, diets like the Mediterranean diet, which is high in fruits, vegetables, whole grains, & healthy fats, have been repeatedly associated with a decreased risk of cancer.

Likewise, plant-based diets that prioritise legumes, nuts, & seeds & limit processed foods can aid in lowering oxidative stress & chronic inflammation. Examining these trends offers helpful advice to anyone wishing to match their diet with cancer prevention techniques.

Making whole, plant-based food consumption a priority is one of the most effective strategies to use nutrition to prevent cancer. A wealth of antioxidants, phytochemicals, vitamins, & minerals found in vegetables, fruits, whole grains, legumes, nuts, & seeds work together to prevent inflammation & cellular damage. For instance, sulforaphane, a substance with strong anti-cancer effects that may prevent tumour growth & encourage the detoxification of carcinogens, is found in cruciferous vegetables like broccoli, kale, & cauliflower. Similarly, anthocyanins, a class of antioxidant that aids in scavenging free radicals & repairing oxidative DNA damage, are abundant in berries. Fibre, which is essential for preserving gut health, controlling insulin levels, & promoting a healthy microbiome—all of which are associated with a lower risk of cancer—is found in whole grains like quinoa, oats, & brown rice.

Particularly in lowering the risk of colorectal cancer, fibre is essential for cancer prevention. Higher fibre consumption may also reduce the risk of ovarian & breast cancers, according to research, possibly by promoting hormone balance & lowering circulating oestrogen levels. The ability of fibre to control insulin &

blood sugar levels may also lower the risk of prostate & pancreatic cancers. Fibre is a versatile tool in the prevention of cancer in all its forms by promoting good gut flora & preserving a healthy digestive system. It promotes regular bowel movements, which aid in the removal of toxins & other dangerous materials from the digestive system. Additionally, fibre serves as a prebiotic, supporting good gut flora that generate butyrate & other short-chain fatty acids. These fatty acids offer an extra line of defence against the growth of tumours because of their anti-inflammatory & anti-carcinogenic properties. A straightforward but effective method for promoting digestive health & reducing the risk of cancer is to consume at least 25 to 30 grammes of fibre per day from a variety of foods, such as fruits, vegetables, & whole grains.

Certain micronutrients & phytochemicals present in plant-based foods, in addition to fibre, provide particular protective advantages. Tomatoes, watermelon, & pink grapefruit contain lycopene, a substance that has been linked to a lower risk of prostate cancer. Its antioxidant qualities may prevent cancer cells from proliferating & aid in the fight against oxidative stress. Similarly, the body converts carotenoids—found in spinach, sweet potatoes, & carrots—into vitamin A & uses them to support normal cell differentiation. The anti-inflammatory & anti-tumor properties of flavonoids, which are present in foods like tea, apples, & onions, highlight the value of a diverse & vibrant diet.

Healthy fats are important, but plant-based foods are the mainstay of a diet that prevents cancer. Flaxseeds, chia seeds, & walnuts, as well as fatty fish like salmon, mackerel, & sardines, contain omega-3 fatty acids, which have been associated with decreased inflammation & a decreased risk of cancer. These fats support immune response regulation, gene expression modulation, & cellular membrane integrity. Conversely, consuming too much saturated & trans fats—which are frequently present in baked goods, fried foods, & fast food—is linked to chronic inflammation & an elevated risk of cancer. A preventive nutrition plan must include both moderation & careful fat source selection.

Limiting or avoiding foods & substances known to increase the risk of cancer is equally important. When cooked, nitrates & nitrites found in processed meats like bacon, sausages, & hot dogs can combine to form carcinogenic compounds. Another important risk factor is alcohol use; even moderate drinking is associated with an increased risk of esophageal, liver, & breast cancers. Although they are not directly carcinogenic, sugary foods & drinks are linked to obesity & insulin resistance, two factors that foster the growth of cancer. Cutting back on these dangerous substances promotes longevity & general health in addition to lowering the risk of cancer.

Drinking the right beverages & staying hydrated are also important in preventing cancer. Drinking water on a regular basis is crucial for preserving cellular health & eliminating toxins, & drinks like coffee & green tea have extra advantages. Green tea may help lower the risk of colorectal, prostate, & breast cancers because it contains catechins, which are strong polyphenols with anti-cancer & antioxidant qualities. Similarly, coffee's high antioxidant content has been linked to a decreased risk of endometrial & liver cancers. A balanced strategy for hydration & cancer prevention involves prioritising water as the main beverage & consuming coffee & green tea in moderation. For example, catechins, a kind of polyphenol with potent antioxidant & anti-cancer effects, are found in green tea. Regular green tea consumption may lower the risk of colorectal, prostate, & breast cancers, according to studies. Similarly, coffee's high antioxidant content has been linked to a lower risk of endometrial & liver cancers when taken in moderation. However, since they can exacerbate inflammation & metabolic dysfunction, drinks that contain a lot of added sugar or artificial sweeteners should be avoided.

Adopting the idea of dietary diversity is a realistic way to adopt a cancer-preventive diet. People can make sure they get a wide range of nutrients that work together to prevent cancer by including a variety of fruits, vegetables, whole grains, & lean proteins in their diet. For example, the Mediterranean diet, which includes moderate amounts of fish & poultry & high amounts of fruits, vegetables, nuts, whole grains, & olive oil, has been repeatedly associated with a lower incidence of cancer. It is a perfect model for cancer prevention because of its focus on plant-based foods, healthy fats, & few processed foods.

Cooking & meal preparation techniques should also be carefully considered. Foods that are grilled, fried, or smoked can release toxic substances like polycyclic aromatic hydrocarbons (PAHs) & heterocyclic amines (HCAs), which are linked to an increased risk of cancer. The production of these carcinogens can be reduced by using healthier cooking methods like baking, boiling, steaming, or stir-frying. Furthermore, adding herbs & spices like ginger, garlic, & turmeric to food not only improves flavour but also gives it anti-inflammatory & anti-cancer qualities.

The amount & timing of food consumption also affect the risk of cancer. Consistently eating large portions or overeating leads to weight gain & obesity, which are major risk factors for a number of cancers, including endometrial, colon, & breast cancers. The potential benefits of intermittent fasting & time-restricted eating, which involve consuming food within a specific window of time, in preventing cancer have drawn attention. These methods may increase insulin sensitivity, lower inflammation, & encourage autophagy & other cellular repair mechanisms that help get rid of damaged cells before they become cancerous.

Notwithstanding the abundance of data demonstrating the protective effects of nutrition against cancer, individual differences must be taken into consideration. Cancer risk is influenced by a number of interrelated factors, including age, genetics, pre-existing medical conditions, & lifestyle decisions. In addition to diet, lifestyle choices like consistent exercise, getting enough sleep, managing stress, & abstaining from tobacco use are important in reducing the risk of cancer. For example, exercise strengthens the immune system & helps control hormones like oestrogen & insulin that are linked to some types of cancer. Good sleep lowers inflammation & promotes cellular repair, which makes the environment less conducive to the growth of cancer. Stress reduction techniques like yoga or meditation can reduce chronic inflammation & enhance general health. People can take a holistic approach to lowering their risk of developing cancer by combining these lifestyle choices with a healthy diet. Dietary recommendations can be more specifically tailored to each person's needs & preferences when healthcare professionals, such as nutritionists or dietitians, are consulted. For example, people who are lactose intolerant may choose calcium-rich plant-based substitutes, & people who are gluten sensitive may consider nutrient-dense, gluten-free grains such as amaranth & quinoa.

It doesn't have to be difficult or restrictive to incorporate these dietary techniques into everyday life. Over time, even small, incremental changes, like choosing whole-grain bread instead of white bread, substituting fresh fruit for sugary snacks, or adding an extra serving of vegetables to meals, can have a big effect. Long-term success in preventing cancer requires developing enduring habits rather than adhering to fad diets. Furthermore, cultivating a healthy relationship with food that places an emphasis on enjoyment & nourishment can improve overall quality of life & adherence to healthy eating habits.

The link between cancer prevention & nutrition is encouraging & empowering. Adopting a balanced, nutrient-rich diet can significantly lower risk & improve general health, even though no one food or nutrient can ensure immunity against cancer. People can take proactive measures to protect their health & live a vibrant, cancer-resistant life by making educated decisions & embracing the protective potential of whole foods.

The Power Of Whole Foods

Whole foods are powerful because of their unmatched capacity to supply a variety of vital nutrients, phytochemicals, & dietary fibre, all of which work together to promote general health & dramatically lower the risk of chronic illnesses like cancer. Natural, unprocessed, or minimally processed whole foods preserve their original nutritional profiles without the harmful effects of refinement, which deplete important vitamins, minerals, & fibre. Particularly rich in antioxidants & phytochemicals, fruits & vegetables fight oxidative stress, which is known to cause cellular damage & the development of cancer. For instance, cruciferous vegetables like broccoli, cauliflower, & Brussels sprouts contain glucosinolates, which activate detoxification enzymes & prevent the growth of cancer cells, while vibrantly coloured vegetables like bell peppers, carrots, & sweet potatoes are high in carotenoids, which boost immune response & shield cells from DNA damage. Anthocyanins & ellagic acid, which are abundant in berries like blueberries, raspberries, & strawberries, counteract free radicals & aid in cellular repair processes. Dietary fibre, which is abundant in whole grains like brown rice, quinoa, oats, & whole wheat, is essential for sustaining a healthy digestive system because it encourages regular bowel movements & a healthy gut microbiome. Short-chain fatty acids, such as butyrate, are produced when gut bacteria ferment fibre. These fatty acids have anti-inflammatory qualities & may offer protection against colorectal cancer. Almonds, walnuts, chia seeds, flaxseeds, & other nuts & seeds provide protein, healthy fats, & micronutrients like vitamin E & selenium that support immunological & cellular integrity. Legumes that promote cell division & repair, such as lentils, chickpeas, & black beans, are also great sources of iron, folate, & plant-based protein. Because of their low glycaemic index & high fibre content, which increase satiety, stabilise blood sugar, & prevent insulin resistance—a condition associated with an increased risk of several cancers—whole foods also naturally regulate energy intake. Whole foods are devoid of trans fats, added sugars, & artificial preservatives, which are found in processed foods & are known to exacerbate oxidative damage & chronic inflammation. Because whole foods are frequently less resource-intensive to produce than highly processed alternatives, eating them promotes a sustainable relationship with the environment in addition to their immediate health benefits. Making meals with whole foods enables people to avoid hidden ingredients that compromise health objectives while incorporating a variety of flavours & textures into their diets. A simple bowl of muesli with fresh berries, nuts & seeds on top, for instance, not only offers a healthy start to the day but also serves as an example of how whole foods are accessible & versatile in everyday life. A key component of preventive healthcare, research continuously shows that diets high in whole foods, like the Mediterranean diet & plant-based eating patterns, are linked to decreased risks of heart disease, diabetes, obesity, & several types of cancer. These dietary patterns strike the perfect balance for long-term health by emphasising the consumption of natural, unprocessed ingredients while reducing the intake of refined carbohydrates, added sugars, & unhealthy fats. Whole foods with anti-inflammatory & immune-modulating qualities, such as turmeric, garlic, & onions, also contain bioactive compounds that strengthen their anti-cancer effects. Aside from being a sensible way to increase nutritional value, including whole foods in the diet also helps protect the body's natural detoxification systems & lower exposure to potentially hazardous additives. People give themselves the power to take charge of their health, guard against chronic illnesses, & maintain a vibrant quality of life over time by selecting whole, nutrient-dense foods over processed ones.

The Role Of Antioxidants & Phytochemicals

Phytochemicals & antioxidants are powerful natural health protectors that play an essential role in warding off chronic diseases like cancer, heart disease, & neurological disorders. Free radicals are unstable molecules that cause oxidative stress & damage cellular components like DNA, proteins, & lipids. These compounds, which are abundant in plant-based foods, work together to neutralise them. Because it causes genetic mutations, chronic inflammation, & the disruption of normal cell signalling pathways, oxidative stress is recognised as a precursor to the development of many cancers. Phytochemicals, which are bioactive substances found only in plants, modulate cellular processes & strengthen the body's natural defences in a variety of indirect ways, in contrast to antioxidants like selenium, beta-carotene, & vitamins C & E, which scavenge free radicals & repair oxidative damage directly. Foods such as berries, green tea, & dark chocolate contain phytochemicals called polyphenols, which have antioxidant & anti-inflammatory effects. This is because they block enzymes & pathways that cause chronic inflammation, which is a characteristic of cancer development. Citrus fruits, apples, onions, & soy are rich in flavonoids, a type of polyphenol that helps protect cells by lowering inflammation, increasing the antioxidant defence system, & even triggering programmed cell death in precancerous cells. Carrots, sweet potatoes, & leafy greens are rich in carotenoids, a group of phytochemicals that do double duty as pigments & antioxidants, preventing DNA damage & promoting healthy cell communication. The tomato carotenoid lycopene has been the subject of substantial research regarding its potential to lower the incidence of breast & prostate cancers through its effects on hormone levels & the inhibition of cancer cell proliferation. Similarly, cruciferous vegetables like broccoli, kale, & Brussels sprouts contain the sulfur-containing phytochemical sulforaphane, which activates detoxification enzymes that aid in the expulsion of carcinogens & the suppression of tumour growth. Antioxidants & phytochemicals not only protect cells from damage, but they also help the immune system function normally, which is critical for preventing cancer by destroying aberrant cells in their early stages. Vitamin C, which is abundant in bell peppers, strawberries, & citrus fruits, helps the body fight off harmful free radicals, boosts white blood cell production, & keeps the skin & mucosal barriers strong, which are its first line of defence against harmful invaders & pollutants. Vitamin E, which is found in abundance in nuts, seeds, & vegetable oils, & vitamin C work together to regenerate & maintain antioxidant activity. It protects cell membranes from oxidative damage. Brazil nuts, shellfish, & whole grains are good sources of selenium, a trace mineral that helps the body produce more glutathione peroxidase & other antioxidant enzymes that protect cells from oxidative damage. Resveratrol, a phytochemical present in red grapes & wine, & curcumin, a turmeric-derived phytochemical, have recently attracted a lot of interest due to their potential to control gene expression & block pathways that contribute to cancer metastasis. Angiogenesis is the process by which tumours create new blood vessels to support their growth. Resveratrol, on the other hand, inhibits this process, essentially depriving cancer cells of nutrients. Conversely, curcumin demonstrates a wide array of anti-cancer actions, including modulating cell cycle progression, increasing treatment sensitivity in cancer cells, & decreasing inflammation & oxidative stress. Rather than taking antioxidants & phytochemicals in isolation, it is best to incorporate them into a varied, nutrient-rich diet for maximum synergy. The complex matrix of bioactive chemicals found in whole foods such as berries, nuts, leafy greens, & spices is thought to enhance their protective effects in ways that are not completely understood. Citrus fruits' vitamin C & flavonoids work together to increase their bioavailability, while avocados & olive oil's fats help the body absorb vegetables' fat-soluble carotenoids. Because of these interdependencies, eating a varied diet is crucial for providing complete protection from oxidative stress & inflammation, as various foods contain different antioxidant & phytochemical profiles that work together. In addition to preventing cancer, these compounds are essential for cardiovascular health because they lower blood pressure, improve endothelial function, & reduce LDL cholesterol oxidation. Antioxidants, such as polyphenols, shield neurones in the brain from free radical damage, which may impede the advancement of cognitive decline associated with ageing & diseases like Alzheimer's. Not all phytochemicals & antioxidants are created equal, & taking too many of them at once might have the opposite effect of what you're hoping for. It is important to maintain a balanced & moderate intake of isolated antioxidants like beta-carotene or vitamin E because excessive amounts of these nutrients have been associated with an increased risk of cancer in some populations. To avoid any potential harm & to work in harmony with the body's natural defences against oxidative stress, it is best to consume these compounds in their whole, unprocessed form. For example, a diet rich in a variety of fruits & vegetables, including bell peppers, spinach, blueberries, & tomatoes, in addition to whole grains, nuts, & green tea, can offer a powerful arsenal of phytochemicals & antioxidants that are specifically designed to combat oxidative damage & promote general well-being. Steaming, for example, is easier on antioxidants than boiling or frying, which can destroy delicate nutrients; both cooking methods contribute to maintaining the compounds' potency. Kimchi, yoghurt, & miso are fermented foods that increase the bioavailability of specific phytochemicals; this highlights the significance of proper preparation methods for getting the most out of these foods. To sum up, phytochemicals & antioxidants are vital partners in the fight for long-term health, providing a holistic & all-natural strategy to ward off cancer & other debilitating conditions. A healthier & more resilient future is within reach when people adopt a plant-based diet that includes a variety of these compounds. By doing so, they can harness their protective power to fight against oxidative stress, inflammation, & cellular damage.

Reducing Cancer Risk with A Balanced Diet

A better grasp of the interconnected nature of nutrition, cellular health, & the immune system is necessary for reducing cancer risk through dietary means. The immune system, hormone balance, & the reduction of chronic inflammation & oxidative stress—two factors associated with cancer development—are all positively impacted by a varied & well-balanced diet. At its core, this strategy revolves around the consumption of nutrient-dense, minimally processed, whole foods. Because of their high vitamin, mineral, fibre, & bioactive compound content, including phytochemicals & antioxidants, fruits & vegetables form the backbone of a cancer-preventive diet. Free radicals are unstable molecules that can damage DNA, cause mutations, & initiate cancerous growths; these components are crucial in neutralising them. Broccoli, Brussels sprouts, & cauliflower are examples of cruciferous vegetables; their glucosinolates, when broken down, produce isothiocyanates, which have anti-carcinogenic & tumor-inhibiting properties. Flavonoids & polyphenols, which are abundant in pomegranates, oranges, & berries, fight oxidative stress & regulate signalling pathways that lead to cell growth or apoptosis, a programmed cell death that stops damaged cells from proliferating.

As an important part of a healthy diet, whole grains should be included because they contain fibre, vitamins,

& phytonutrients. Quinoa, oats, & brown rice are examples of whole grains that can aid in blood sugar regulation & insulin resistance reduction, both of which are associated with a decreased risk of developing breast & colon cancers, among others. The fibre in whole grains helps keep the digestive tract healthy in a number of ways, including encouraging regular bowel movements, decreasing the amount of time carcinogens spend in contact with the intestinal lining, & encouraging a diverse gut microbiome. However, this microbiome also produces butyrate & other short-chain fatty acids that have anti-inflammatory & anti-carcinogenic characteristics. A well-rounded diet must also include legumes like black beans, chickpeas, & lentils because they are low in saturated fat & provide protein & fibre. In addition, they supply resistant starch, a carbohydrate that prebiotically feeds good gut bacteria & amplifies their anti-inflammatory & anti-cancer potential.

Essential to any diet aimed at warding off cancer are the healthy fats found in foods like avocados, nuts, seeds, & fatty fish. Omega-3 fatty acids, which are abundant in walnuts, mackerel, & salmon, have been the subject of substantial research due to their anti-inflammatory & anti-angiogenic qualities. These lipids help create an unfriendly environment for cancer cells by lowering systemic inflammation & bolstering the structural integrity of cell membranes. Fried foods, processed snacks, & baked goods are rich in saturated & trans fats, which are linked to inflammation & an increased risk of cancer, including colorectal & prostate cancers. In order to reduce the likelihood of cancer, it is important to eat a variety of healthy fats while limiting the consumption of unhealthy ones.

Another important factor in preventing cancer is consuming protein-rich foods as part of a healthy diet. To build cells & keep the immune system working, eat lean proteins like chicken, fish, tofu, & lentils instead of processed & red meats. The World Health Organisation has classified processed meats such as sausages, bacon, & hot dogs as carcinogens. This is because these meats contain a high concentration of nitrates & nitrites, which can transform into harmful compounds when cooked. An elevated risk of colorectal & pancreatic cancers has been associated with the production of heterocyclic amines (HCAs) & polycyclic aromatic hydrocarbons (PAHs) by red meats when they are overcooked or eaten in large quantities. To lessen these risks & add fibre & phytochemicals to your diet, try plant-based protein alternatives like edamame, chickpeas, & lentils.

Many people fail to remember that staying hydrated is a crucial part of a healthy diet when it comes to preventing cancer. It is important to drink enough of water to support digestive processes, flush out toxins, & keep cells healthy. Green tea & coffee, which are rich in antioxidants & polyphenols, have been linked to a lower risk of cancer, particularly colorectal & liver cancers. But you should cut back on sugary drinks & alcohol because they make you fat & throw your metabolism for a loop, which increases your chances of getting cancer. Particularly associated with an increased risk of breast, liver, & esophageal cancers, alcohol is a recognised carcinogen. To maximise the protective effects of a healthy diet, drink alcohol in moderation or not at all.

A well-rounded diet has the ability to fight cancer, & spices & herbs play an additional role in this. Curcumin, the active ingredient in turmeric, has anti-inflammatory & cancer-fighting properties. While ginger's anti-inflammatory & antioxidant qualities may lower the risk of gastrointestinal cancers, garlic's sulphur compounds enhance the immune system's capacity to neutralise carcinogens. Meals are made more appetising & provide an extra nutritional shield against cancer when a variety of these natural flavour enhancers are used.

Cancer risk is also affected by meal timing & portion sizes. Obesity & weight gain are major risk factors for many types of cancer, including breast, endometrial, & esophageal cancers, among others. The possibility that time-restricted eating, also known as intermittent fasting, can improve metabolic health & cellular repair mechanisms like autophagy has attracted a lot of attention. Cancer initiation & progression can be slowed by following these dietary practices, which give the body enough time to repair & eliminate damaged cells.

An additional important component in lowering the risk of cancer is cooking techniques. Particularly when meats are subjected to high temperatures, methods like smoking, frying, & grilling can produce carcinogenic compounds like PAHs & HCAs. Cooking foods in healthier ways, like steaming, boiling, baking, or stir-frying, keeps their nutrients intact & reduces the formation of unhealthy substances. To further decrease the formation of these compounds, herbs, citrus juices, or vinegar marinating meats before cooking can result in safer & more nutritious meals.

To make sure the body gets a diverse range of nutrients, phytochemicals, & antioxidants, a balanced diet should include a variety of foods. Reduced cancer risks have been associated with dietary patterns such as the Mediterranean diet, which includes plenty of fruits & vegetables, whole grains, healthy fats, & lean proteins. A sustainable & healthful diet can be modelled after this one, which emphasises plant-based foods, olive oil, & moderate fish consumption. Similarly, there are significant benefits to reducing chronic inflammation & oxidative stress by adopting a plant-based diet that emphasises nuts, seeds, legumes, & whole grains while reducing reliance on animal products.

Although there is evidence that a healthy diet can help reduce the risk of cancer, it is important to remember that everyone is different. Diet is just one factor among many that affect cancer risk factors, which also include heredity, prior health issues, & lifestyle choices. Under the guidance of medical experts, personalised nutrition can assist in customising food plans to meet specific requirements. For those who can't digest lactose, there are plant-based milks that are fortified with calcium.

Gluten-free grains, such as quinoa & amaranth, can help those who are sensitive to gluten.

Adopting sustainable, pleasurable eating habits that prioritise long-term health is the ultimate goal of reducing cancer risk through a balanced diet. Over time, little adjustments like swapping out sugary snacks for fresh fruit, opting for whole-grain alternatives to refined grains, or increasing the amount of vegetables in meals can add up to a big difference. One way people can take charge of their health & lower their risk of cancer is by eating more whole, nutrient-dense foods & less processed & nasty ones. An effective diet that nourishes the body & protects against the development of chronic diseases, including cancer, can be built upon a combination of mindful eating practices & a diverse diet rich in nutrients.

Foods To Limit Or Avoid For Optimal Health

To keep one's health in tip-top shape, one must avoid consuming foods that raise the risk of chronic diseases, inflammation, cancer, heart disease, & diabetes, among others. Highly processed & ultra-processed foods are heavy of refined sugars, bad fats, sodium, & artificial additives, making them a leading cause. The World Health Organisation (WHO) has classified processed meats like bacon, sausages, hot dogs, & deli meats as Group 1 carcinogens, which is especially worrisome. The nitrates & nitrites found in these meats have the potential to transform into carcinogenic substances when they are cooked & processed. Heterocyclic amines

(HCAs) & polycyclic aromatic hydrocarbons (PAHs) are carcinogens, & eating red meat on a regular basis, especially when cooked to high temperatures (grilling, frying, or broiling), increases the risk of cancer, especially colorectal cancer. Obesity, insulin resistance, & metabolic syndrome are major risk factors for chronic diseases like diabetes & certain cancers. Sugary beverages, such as soda, energy drinks, & sweetened fruit juices, contribute to these conditions. Furthermore, trans fats, which are present in fried fast food, baked goods, margarine, & partially hydrogenated oils, are associated with elevated inflammation & an increased risk of cardiovascular disease.

Foods heavy in added sugars are another group to cut back on because they cause inflammation throughout the body, throw off hormone balance, & add extra pounds to your waistline. Type 2 diabetes, cancers associated with obesity, & cardiovascular conditions are just some of the diseases that can flourish in an atmosphere where these effects are present. Prepackaged & canned foods are a major source of sodium, which can cause high blood pressure & increase the risk of cardiovascular disease & stroke. The gut microbiota can be changed by artificial sweeteners, which are promoted as healthier alternatives to sugar. This change could lead to metabolic dysfunction. Even moderate alcohol consumption has been associated with an increased risk of several malignancies, including those of the oesophagus, breast, & liver. Tobacco & alcohol have a multiplicative effect that increases the dangers already present, making carcinogenesis much more likely.

In addition to avoiding or reducing your intake of fried & highly charred foods, it is wise to steer clear of foods that are cooked in a way that produces acrylamides & advanced glycation end-products (AGEs), which are compounds that promote inflammation & oxidative stress. White bread, pasta, & pastries are examples of refined grains; they lack the fibre & nutrients found in whole grains & cause insulin & blood sugar levels to spike quickly, which can lead to diabetes & some cancers. On the other hand, whole grains aid with blood sugar regulation & intestinal health by providing necessary fibre & nutrients. Worries about the carcinogenic & allergenic properties of artificial food dyes, preservatives, & flavour enhancers have been voiced in relation to snack foods, candies, & fast food; however, in certain instances, more research is required.

Cutting back or cutting out these foods isn't about starving yourself; it's about intentionally choosing to eat more whole, less processed foods. Creating a dietary pattern that supports long-term health, resilience against chronic diseases, & overall vitality can be achieved by reducing exposure to harmful substances. Substituting fresh fruit for processed snacks, water or herbal tea for sugary drinks, & lean proteins & whole grains for processed foods can all add up to big changes in your health over time. People can empower themselves to live healthier, more balanced lives by raising awareness & actively limiting harmful foods.

Building A Sustainable & Healthy Meal Plan

The foundation of long-term health & disease prevention is developing a sustainable & healthful eating plan that promotes physical vitality & complies with ethical & environmental standards. Numerous nutrient-dense foods are included in a balanced meal plan to satisfy each person's energy needs & promote general wellness. Prioritise whole, unprocessed foods such as fruits, vegetables, whole grains, lean meats, & healthy fats first. These foods minimise added sugars, bad fats, & sodium while providing important macronutrients, fibre, vitamins, & minerals. Lean meats, fish, eggs, legumes, tofu, & other plant-based sources of protein should be taken into account. Make sure you consume enough amino acids without consuming too much saturated fat. Consume a diverse range of fruits & vegetables every day to optimise your intake of antioxidants & phytochemicals, which help lower oxidative stress & inflammation & guard against chronic illnesses. Slow-digesting carbohydrates & fibre from whole grains like quinoa, brown rice, & oats help to maintain stable blood sugar levels & support digestive health.

Omega-3 fatty acids & other compounds necessary for brain health & lowering systemic inflammation are found in healthy fats like those in avocados, nuts, seeds, & fatty fish. The risk of heart disease & some types of cancer is also decreased by reducing trans fats & excessive saturated fats. By promoting sustainable farming methods, meal planning that incorporates locally grown & seasonal produce not only improves flavour & nutrient density but also lessens its environmental impact. Water is the best beverage for preserving cellular health & promoting metabolic processes, so hydration is equally important. While sugar-filled beverages & high-calorie options should be avoided, herbal teas & unsweetened beverages can provide variety.

When creating a sustainable meal plan, structure is essential. Maintain portion sizes that correspond with each person's activity level & objectives while balancing meals to include a source of protein, complex carbs, & healthy fats. A mixed greens salad with grilled chicken, quinoa & a lemon-tahini dressing could be served for lunch, & muesli with fresh berries & nuts could be served for breakfast. Keep snacks like sliced veggies with hummus, yoghurt, or a handful of almonds on hand for mindful eating in between meals, & think about serving roasted salmon with steamed broccoli & a baked sweet potato for dinner. Meal plans can accommodate dietary restrictions, cultural customs, & individual preferences by adhering to the concepts of moderation & variety, which promotes consistency & enjoyment.

Adaptability & readiness are also key components of sustainability. When life gets hectic, meal planning & batch cooking can save time & lessen the temptation to make unhealthy choices. Quick & wholesome meals are always accessible with easy tactics like pre-cooking grains & proteins or keeping chopped vegetables & prepared sauces on hand. Whether ordering in or dining out, selecting balanced options—like grilled or steamed foods, whole grains, & entrees high in vegetables—helps keep in line with a healthy eating pattern. Over time, flexibility makes the plan more enjoyable & realistic by allowing for occasional indulgences.

Last but not least, a sustainable diet plan takes into account its wider effects in addition to personal health. A more environmentally conscious approach is supported by minimising food waste through careful portion planning, freezing leftovers, & repurposing ingredients into new meals. Several times a week, eating plant-based meals can help reduce carbon footprints & support international initiatives to encourage environmental stewardship. People can promote long-term adherence to healthy habits & build resilience against chronic diseases like diabetes, cancer, & cardiovascular conditions by seeing meal plans as flexible frameworks rather than strict rules. They can also help create a more sustainable planet.

This strategy combines sustainability, health, & practicality, giving people the confidence & drive to sustain long-term, nourishing eating habits.

CHAPTER 2: PHYSICAL ACTIVITY AS A SHIELD

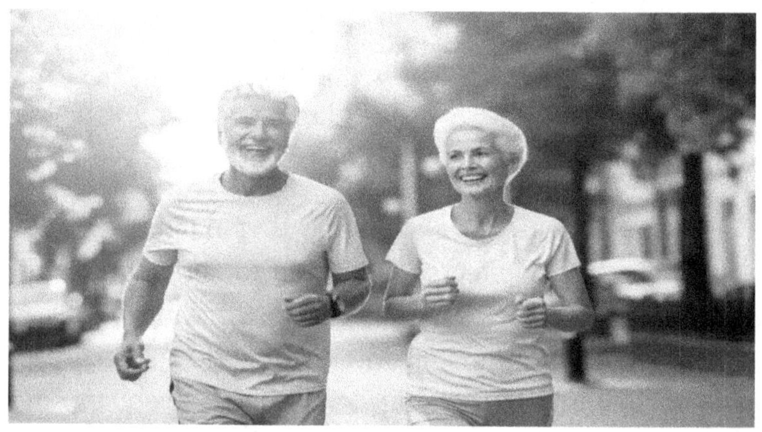

Exercise greatly improves general health & quality of life while acting as a potent barrier against a wide range of chronic illnesses, such as cancer, heart disease, diabetes, & obesity. Frequent exercise enhances metabolic efficiency, builds bone & muscle mass, & improves cardiovascular fitness, all of which actively reduce the risk of disease. Its capacity to control hormone levels, such as insulin & oestrogen, is one of its most important functions. This regulation can affect the occurrence of hormone-sensitive cancers, such as endometrial & breast cancers. Additionally, oxidative stress & systemic inflammation—both of which are connected to cellular damage & carcinogenesis—are decreased by physical activity. Because obesity is a known risk factor for a number of cancers, including colorectal, pancreatic, & kidney cancers, exercise is crucial for maintaining a healthy weight in addition to its physiological advantages.

Running, cycling, & swimming are examples of aerobic exercises that enhance circulation & heart health by more effectively supplying oxygen & nutrients to tissues & promoting the elimination of waste. Conversely, resistance training increases bone density & muscle strength, which are essential for preserving function & lowering the risk of osteoporosis, particularly in older populations. Regular exercise also promotes mental health by lowering stress, anxiety, & depression—all of which can impair general wellbeing & immune system performance. There is a strong link between mental & physical health because lower stress levels strengthen the body's defences against illness by reducing inflammation & enhancing cellular repair processes.

When creating a successful physical activity program, the frequency, duration, & intensity of exercise are important considerations. At least 150 minutes of moderate-intensity aerobic exercise or 75 minutes of vigorous-intensity exercise per week, along with two or more days of muscle-strengthening activities, are advised by current guidelines. But over time, even modest, regular efforts—like taking the stairs, walking, or gardening—can add up to big advantages. Including physical activity in daily routines, such as walking or cycling to work, taking part in group fitness classes, or discovering fun pastimes like dancing or hiking, can also promote adherence.

The protective benefits of physical activity also include increased immune system effectiveness. Exercise increases the flow of immune cells, which makes it easier for them to identify & eliminate infections or aberrant cells, like cancerous cells in their early stages. Additionally, exercise helps control insulin sensitivity & blood sugar levels, two variables that are directly associated with a lower risk of cancers like colorectal & pancreatic cancer. Exercise aids in lowering chronic inflammation, which creates an environment that is conducive to tumour growth, by lowering inflammation markers such as C-reactive protein (CRP).

Physical activity is also essential for cancer survivors' recuperation & recurrence prevention. Frequent exercise has been demonstrated to alleviate fatigue, elevate mood, & restore strength, all of which greatly improve quality of life both during & after treatment. Oncology care has begun to incorporate customised physical activity programs for survivors, highlighting the many advantages of maintaining an active lifestyle.

In the end, physical activity is an essential component of a preventive lifestyle that strengthens the body & mind against disease, & it goes beyond simply keeping fit. People can fully utilise physical activity as a protective barrier that promotes resilience, vitality, & long-term health by incorporating movement into their daily lives & realising its many advantages.

The Science Of Exercise In Cancer Prevention

A fascinating nexus of physiology, biochemistry, & epidemiology, the science of exercise in cancer prevention shows how regular physical activity is a powerful way to lower the risk of developing cancer. Exercise has a profound effect on hormone regulation, which is just one of the many ways it affects the body. Increased cell proliferation & the development of cancer are linked to elevated levels of insulin & insulin-like growth factors (IGFs); regular exercise helps control these hormones by enhancing glucose metabolism & insulin sensitivity. Exercise also lowers levels of androgens & oestrogen in the blood, which are linked to hormone-sensitive cancers like prostate, ovarian, & breast cancers. Exercise reduces one of the main pathways through which cancers grow by preserving hormonal balance. Furthermore, exercise promotes the synthesis of myokines, which are proteins released during muscle contractions & have anti-inflammatory & tumor-suppressive qualities.

Exercise improves immune function at the cellular level by boosting the circulation of T cells, natural killer cells, & macrophages—all of which are essential for detecting & eliminating precancerous & cancerous cells. Frequent exercise also encourages effective DNA repair processes, which lowers the risk of genetic alterations that could result in the development of tumours. Additionally, exercise reduces oxidative stress &

chronic inflammation, two factors that are strongly linked to the development & spread of cancer. This is accomplished by increasing antioxidant defences & decreasing inflammatory markers like interleukin-6 (IL-6) & tumour necrosis factor-alpha (TNF-α).

These biological processes are regularly supported by epidemiological research, which shows a direct link between physical activity & a lower risk of cancer. For example, those who regularly exercise moderately to vigorously have a much lower risk of endometrial, breast, & colorectal cancers than those who are sedentary. Because the protective effects are dose-dependent, the benefits of exercise are increased with increased frequency, intensity, & duration. It has been demonstrated that even small amounts of physical activity, like 30 minutes a day of brisk walking, significantly lower the risk of cancer, highlighting the accessibility of exercise as a preventive strategy.

Additionally, exercise is essential for keeping a healthy weight, which is a key component in preventing cancer. Adipokines like leptin, which are produced by excess body fat, can encourage the growth of tumours & are a cause of chronic inflammation. Exercise not only aids in weight loss but also lowers visceral fat, a particularly dangerous kind of fat associated with a higher risk of cancer. Exercise also promotes metabolic health by lowering blood pressure, improving cardiovascular efficiency, & improving lipid profiles—all of which help to create a strong internal environment that inhibits the growth of cancer.

Physical activity has been demonstrated to reduce the risk of recurrence & increase survival rates in cancer survivorship, extending the science of exercise beyond prevention. This is especially true for survivors of prostate, colorectal, & breast cancer, where exercise after diagnosis is linked to improved outcomes. Frequent exercise improves psychological well-being by lowering anxiety & depression & helps lessen the negative effects of cancer treatments, such as fatigue, muscle loss, & decreased bone density.

Exercise is a key component of preventive health strategies because of the dynamic & complex mechanisms through which it protects against cancer. Physical activity encourages people to take proactive measures to protect their health by improving immune surveillance, controlling hormones, lowering inflammation, & fostering metabolic health. Exercise's role in preventing cancer will only solidify as more research reveals the complexities of how it interacts with cellular & systemic processes, highlighting the importance of making movement a top priority in leading a healthy lifestyle.

Types Of Physical Activity & Their Benefits

A variety of movements that work the body's muscles are included in physical activity, & each has unique advantages for general health & wellbeing. Numerous health advantages, such as increased muscular strength, improved flexibility, decreased risk of chronic diseases,

& improved cardiovascular health, can result from participating in different forms of physical activity.

Running, cycling, swimming, & brisk walking are examples of aerobic exercise (also known as endurance activities) that raise heart rates & increase cardiovascular system performance. Frequent aerobic exercise improves lung & heart health, helps control weight, & lowers the risk of type 2 diabetes, heart disease, & stroke. Aerobic exercise has also been associated with a decreased risk of anxiety & depression as well as enhanced cognitive function.

CDC

Strength Training (Resistance Exercise): This type of exercise involves using weights, resistance bands, & bodyweight exercises (such as squats & push-ups) to build & maintain muscle mass. This kind of exercise improves functional fitness, supports bone density, raises metabolism, & builds muscle strength & endurance—all of which make daily tasks easier. Strength training has also been linked to better brain health, including a lower risk of cognitive decline & enhanced cognitive function.

The New York Post

Exercises for Flexibility: Yoga, Pilates, & other stretching techniques help to increase the range of motion in the muscles & joints. Frequent flexibility exercises improve posture, ease tense muscles, lower the chance of injury, & encourage relaxation. A fitness regimen that includes flexibility exercises can also enhance balance & coordination, which will enhance physical performance in general.

Exercises for Balance: Tai Chi, one-legged standing, & yoga poses that emphasise balance improve coordination & stability. For older adults, improving balance is especially crucial because it lowers their risk of falls & the injuries they cause. Exercises for balance also work the core muscles, which improves posture & allows for more functional movement.

Exercise that alternates short bursts of intense activity with rest or low-intensity exercise is called high-intensity interval training, or HIIT. It has been demonstrated that HIIT raises metabolic rate, increases calorie burn, & improves cardiovascular fitness. Compared to conventional steady-state aerobic exercise, it is an effective method of obtaining notable health benefits in a shorter period of time.

Low-Impact Activities: Cardiovascular exercises that put less strain on the joints include swimming, cycling, & elliptical machine use. These exercises provide a way to remain active while lowering the risk of joint strain & are appropriate for people with joint issues or those recuperating from injuries.

Functional Training: This method improves the body's capacity to carry out daily tasks by using exercises that replicate natural movements. Enhancing strength, balance, & coordination through functional training lowers the chance of injury & increases general physical fitness.

Comprehensive health benefits, such as better cardiovascular health, increased muscular strength, improved flexibility, improved balance, & a lower risk of chronic diseases, can result from incorporating a range of these physical activities into a regular exercise regimen. To maintain consistency & attain the best possible health results, it's critical to select enjoyable activities that are appropriate for each person's level of fitness.

Designing A Fitness Routine For Your Needs

In order to create a fitness regimen that works for you, you must carefully balance a number of elements, each of which is intended to enhance a different facet of your physical health & wellbeing. Your objectives, present level of fitness, & any physical restrictions or health issues you may have are all taken into consideration when creating a fitness program. Determine your main fitness goals first, such as weight loss, muscle growth, cardiovascular health improvement, flexibility improvement, or general strength & endurance gains. Finding the exercises that will best help you reach your goals is the next step after defining them. For instance, if you want to lose weight, adding aerobic activities like swimming, cycling, or running can help you burn calories & strengthen your heart. To maintain muscle mass & increase metabolism, strength training should be included. Resistance training, which uses free weights, machines, or bodyweight exercises like squats & push-ups to target different muscle groups, should be the mainstay of your regimen if your goal is to gain muscle. Yoga, Pilates, or consistent stretching exercises are crucial for flexibility & mobility in order to preserve & improve joint health, avoid injuries, & increase general mobility. To enhance coordination & reduce the risk of falls, particularly as you age, balance exercises like Tai Chi or basic balance drills should be incorporated. Intensity & duration are also important aspects of a fitness regimen. To prevent overtraining & give your body time to recover, your routine should include a combination of low-, moderate-, & high-intensity exercises. High-Intensity Interval Training (HIIT) is a quick & efficient way to increase endurance, burn fat, & improve cardiovascular health. For people who feel uncomfortable during high-impact activities or to protect their joints, low-impact exercises like swimming or cycling can be included. Strength training should focus on gradually increasing resistance to continue building strength, with enough rest in between to allow muscles to grow & recover. Depending on your level of fitness, cardiovascular exercises should be modified. As your stamina increases, you should progressively increase the duration & intensity of your workouts. Additionally, to avoid injury, increase flexibility, & lessen muscle soreness, make sure your fitness regimen incorporates appropriate warm-up & cool-down phases. Consistency is another key component of a well-rounded fitness regimen; try to get in exercise most days of the week, focussing on various muscle groups & switching between cardiovascular, strength, & flexibility training. To get the most out of your routine, nutritional support is just as crucial. Your workouts & recuperation will be fuelled by a well-balanced diet that contains healthy fats for heart & joint health, protein for muscle repair, & carbohydrates for energy. Because it promotes joint health, muscle function, & overall performance, hydration is essential. It's critical to modify your exercise regimen if you have a medical condition or injury & to speak with a healthcare provider or fitness expert to prevent making matters worse. The secret to creating a fitness regimen that suits you is to make it both fun & sustainable. To stay motivated & keep making progress towards improved health & fitness, regularly review your objectives & accomplishments. You should also be willing to modify your regimen as your body changes.

Staying Active: Tips For Busy Lifestyles

Although leading a busy life can make staying active difficult, doing so is crucial for preserving one's physical & mental well-being. The secret to striking this balance is making exercise a priority & introducing it into daily activities in tiny, doable ways. Instead of planning hour-long workouts that could seem overwhelming or impossible to fit into a busy schedule, concentrate on shorter, more intense sessions that yield the most results in a shorter amount of time. An outstanding choice is High-Intensity Interval Training (HIIT), which provides significant cardiovascular & fat-burning advantages in as little as 20 to 30 minutes. Additionally, you can stay active during the time you would normally spend running errands or commuting. Your daily activity level can be influenced by parking farther from your destination, walking or cycling to work, or using the stairs rather than the lift. Scheduling brief but regular breaks throughout the day can help people who prefer more structured workouts avoid burnout & boost their energy levels. It can also be beneficial to incorporate movement into routine tasks, like performing lunges while cooking or squats while brushing your teeth. Furthermore, staying active doesn't have to be done alone. By participating in social activities that require physical activity, like team sports or walking groups, exercise can become less of a chore & more of an enjoyable social occasion. Another crucial factor for maintaining an active lifestyle in the face of a hectic schedule is flexibility. Rigid schedules that leave little time for exercise make it difficult for many people to maintain an active lifestyle. However, you can find innovative ways to incorporate exercise into your routine by staying adaptable & embracing a mindset that values physical activity as a kind of self-care. Maybe this entails taking a quick walk during your lunch break or getting up fifteen minutes earlier for a quick yoga session. You can effectively stay active even when life seems overwhelming by changing the way you approach fitness & paying attention to how you incorporate movement into your everyday routine. Additionally, maintaining motivation & creating momentum can be achieved by establishing reasonable goals & acknowledging minor accomplishments along the way. Celebrate the little victories, whether they are boosting your endurance, increasing your flexibility, or just maintaining a regular exercise schedule, rather than concentrating only on long-term results like weight loss or muscle gain. You'll stay on course & inspired to keep finding time for exercise in your hectic schedule thanks to this encouraging feedback. It's crucial to understand that maintaining an active lifestyle doesn't always necessitate frequenting the gym or doing strenuous exercise. Dancing, gardening, & even housework can all be equally beneficial for encouraging physical activity & improving general health. Asking for help from others is another useful tactic. For extra accountability, think about joining a fitness group or finding a workout partner if you struggle to maintain an exercise regimen on your own. On days when you might otherwise skip a workout, having someone to share the experience with can help you stay motivated & give you the necessary encouragement. In the end, maintaining an active lifestyle while juggling a busy schedule requires prioritising exercise, moving with flexibility, & figuring out how to incorporate physical activity into everyday activities. By doing this, you not only enhance your general health but also your energy, mood, & productivity, enabling you to confidently face even the busiest days. Maintaining an active lifestyle has numerous advantages, impacting everything from emotional fortitude to mental clarity, & the time & effort put into making fitness a priority pays off in the long run. Keep in mind that consistency is crucial as you try out various methods to fit movement into your day.

Your life can change for the better over time with even little spurts of activity.

Overcoming Barriers To Regular Exercise

One of the most important parts of living an active, healthy life is overcoming obstacles to regular exercise, particularly in the fast-paced world of today where motivation, time, & other issues can easily get in the way of the desire to maintain an active lifestyle. Lack of time is one of the most frequent obstacles people encounter, & it frequently results from hectic schedules full of social, familial, & professional obligations. However, by changing one's perspective to emphasise physical activity as an essential component of a balanced lifestyle, this obstacle can be lessened. It can be beneficial to reframe exercise as a kind of self-care & personal investment rather than as an extra chore to fit into an already hectic day. Regular exercise has many advantages, such as better mental clarity, better emotional regulation, decreased stress, & improved physical health, all of which can help you handle the demands of a busy day. People can overcome the time barrier by establishing reasonable goals, segmenting workouts into shorter, easier-to-manage sessions, & making exercise an essential part of their everyday routine. For example, using circuit training or high-intensity interval training (HIIT) can offer effective full-body workouts in as little as 20 to 30 minutes, making them more convenient to fit into a busy schedule. Combining exercise with other everyday routines, like taking active breaks during the day, walking or cycling to work, or taking the stairs rather than the lift, is another beneficial tactic. This enables people to maintain their level of activity without needing to devote more time outside of their regular obligations. Lack of motivation is another significant obstacle to consistent exercise, & it can result from a number of things, including not feeling "in the mood" to work out, boredom with monotonous routines, or a sense of not making any progress. Although motivation can frequently change depending on outside factors, it's important to understand that motivation by itself isn't always sufficient to maintain a regular exercise schedule. Developing a sense of discipline & dedication to fitness, even on days when motivation is low, is crucial to overcoming this. This obstacle can be addressed by establishing a disciplined exercise program & holding oneself accountable, whether through goal-setting, self-monitoring, or enlisting the assistance of a workout partner. Furthermore, exercise can be made more pleasurable & long-lasting by emphasising intrinsic motivation—that is, the joy & fulfilment that come from movement itself—instead of depending on extrinsic rewards like muscle growth or weight loss. Trying out new fitness classes, dancing, hiking, swimming, & other forms of physical activity can also help keep things interesting & fun & keep boredom from becoming a deterrent. Physical restrictions or health issues, such as chronic pain, injuries, or ailments like arthritis or heart disease, which can make movement uncomfortable or even painful, are another major obstacle to regular exercise. Even though these restrictions can be difficult, they shouldn't be viewed as insurmountable barriers. To create a safe & efficient exercise program that meets their individual needs, people must speak with medical professionals or fitness specialists. Low-impact activities like swimming, cycling, or yoga, for instance, can help people with joint pain because they can improve strength & cardiovascular health without placing an excessive amount of strain on the joints. Specific exercises that increase strength & flexibility may help reduce pain & enhance general function for people with back pain or other musculoskeletal conditions. As you gradually increase your strength & endurance over time, it's critical to pay attention to your body & respect its limits. Regular exercise can also be significantly hampered by mental health issues like anxiety, depression, or low self-esteem. Exercise has been shown to be a successful strategy for addressing these problems because it increases endorphins & serotonin, elevates mood, & increases energy. However, it can be hard for people with mental health issues to find the motivation or drive to work out, especially when they're feeling depressed or uninterested. To gradually reintroduce movement into the daily routine in such situations, it's crucial to start small & set attainable goals, like going for a 10-minute walk or doing a quick stretching session. It is beneficial to highlight the positive mental & emotional effects of exercise in addition to its physical advantages, such as stress reduction & the sense of achievement that comes from finishing a workout. In order to overcome obstacles to exercise, social support is essential because it can offer encouragement, accountability, & motivation. Social interaction can make physical activity more fun & help people stick to their fitness goals, whether they are working out with a friend, joining a fitness group, or playing a team sport. Even when personal motivation wanes, group fitness challenges, online communities, or exercise classes can offer the structure & support required to stay on course. Lack of knowledge or comprehension about effective exercise is another frequent obstacle. The thought of exercising can be intimidating to many people, particularly if they are not familiar with the right methods or tools. As a result, people may avoid exercising because they are frustrated, hurt, or lack confidence. To get past this obstacle, it's critical to look for trustworthy information sources, such as fitness courses, personal trainers, internet resources, or instructional videos, in order to gain confidence & understand the basics of exercise. People can feel more at ease & capable in their fitness journey by beginning with easy, beginner-friendly exercises & progressively moving on to more complex routines. Additionally, maintaining long-term success & avoiding burnout or injury requires an awareness of the significance of rest, recuperation, & healthy eating. Exercise can also be hampered by environmental factors, such as a lack of a gym, equipment, or safe outdoor areas, especially for people who live in urban or low-income areas. In these situations, it's crucial to look into alternate workouts that call for little to no equipment, like bodyweight exercises (like lunges, squats, & push-ups) or outdoor pursuits like hiking or running. A variety of options for at-home workouts can also be obtained by using fitness applications, YouTube tutorials, or online workout programs. For those looking for a more structured fitness experience, parks, community programs, or nearby recreation centres may provide reasonably priced options. Focussing on free alternatives, like jogging, walking, or bodyweight exercises, can help people with limited funds maintain a regular exercise routine without having to buy pricey gym memberships or equipment. Lastly, people may find it difficult to maintain a consistent exercise regimen due to irrational expectations & all-or-nothing thinking. Many people give up completely because they expect quick results or get disheartened when they don't see quick progress. It is crucial to adopt a more adaptable, caring approach to exercise & set reasonable, attainable goals in order to get past this obstacle. People should prioritise consistency & long-term sustainability over striving for perfection. It's critical to understand that obstacles & setbacks are normal & shouldn't be interpreted as failures. People are more likely to stick with regular exercise & see long-lasting benefits if they adopt a mindset that prioritises progress over perfection & have patience with the process. Although overcoming obstacles to consistent exercise is not always simple, an active lifestyle can be established & maintained in spite of these difficulties with perseverance, ingenuity, & a readiness to change.

CHAPTER 3: THE IMPORTANCE OF MENTAL WELLNESS

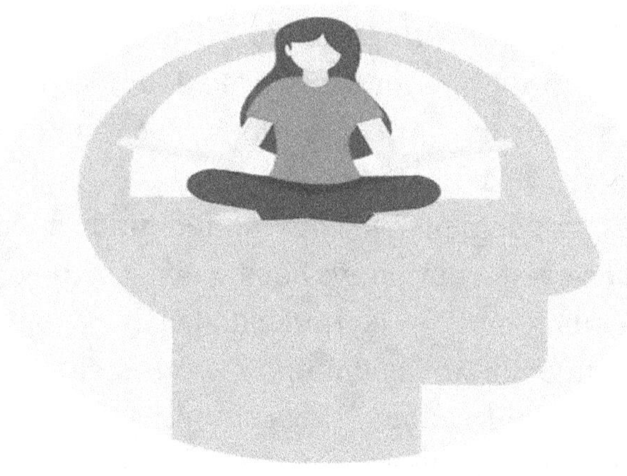

One of the most important—yet frequently disregarded—aspects of general health & wellbeing is mental wellness. It is all too easy for people to disregard their mental health in a society that constantly expects more of them, whether through employment, social expectations, family obligations, or personal objectives. It is impossible to overestimate the significance of mental wellness since it is fundamental to how people view the world, cope with stress, relate to others, & deal with the difficulties that life invariably brings. Every aspect of human life is impacted by mental wellness, including social interactions, physical health, emotional control, & cognitive function. It includes a wide range of social, psychological, & emotional well-being elements that collectively affect people's thoughts, feelings, & behaviours. The capacity to manage everyday stressors, work efficiently, contribute significantly to society, & uphold wholesome relationships are all aspects of mental wellness. Fundamentally, mental wellness involves developing resilience, self-awareness, & balance—all of which are critical for negotiating life's challenges. Understanding the profound effects of mental wellness on both individuals & society at large is crucial to appreciating its significance. Strong mental health makes it easier for people to cope with stress, prevent depressing thoughts, & bounce back from setbacks. Even in the face of hardship, mental wellness can enable people to think critically, make wise decisions, & keep a positive attitude. However, when mental health is impaired, it can show up in a variety of ways, ranging from mood disorders like depression & anxiety to more severe conditions like schizophrenia or bipolar disorder. A person's ability to function in daily life can be severely hampered by these mental health issues, which can also have an impact on relationships with friends, family, & coworkers as well as impede personal, academic, or professional growth. Additionally, mental health issues frequently affect not just the individual dealing with them but also their community & society at large. Poor mental health, for instance, can result in physical health issues like high blood pressure, heart disease, & compromised immune function, as well as decreased productivity & absenteeism from work. Therefore, addressing mental wellness is a matter of both personal self-care & larger societal responsibility. Developing a range of coping mechanisms that can be used during stressful situations, adversity, or emotional upheaval is part of a comprehensive approach to mental wellness. Exercise, mindfulness, meditation, & getting professional help when necessary are common strategies for preserving mental wellness, though different people may find different approaches to be more successful. For example, practicing mindfulness helps people stay in the present & become more self-aware, which makes it possible for them to spot when their thoughts are out of control & take appropriate action to refocus them. Additionally, meditation has several positive effects on mental health, ranging from improving focus & concentration to lowering anxiety & depression. Another effective strategy for preserving mental health is physical activity, which has been demonstrated to lower stress, elevate mood, & enhance cognitive function by releasing endorphins & other neurochemicals. Regular exercise, whether it be yoga, running, walking, or other sports, can help people feel in control of their mental health & develop resilience when faced with obstacles. Additionally, getting professional help—whether in the form of therapy, counselling, or medication—can give people the skills & direction they need to successfully manage mental health issues. Overcoming mental health issues can occasionally call for the assistance of qualified professionals who can provide evidence-based treatment options in addition to self-care routines & coping strategies. Dispelling the stigmas attached to mental health issues is one of the most important parts of fostering mental wellness. Too long, mental health problems have been stigmatised &

kept quiet, & many people are reluctant to get treatment out of fear of being misunderstood or judged. In addition to keeping people from getting the care they require, this stigma feeds negative stereotypes about mental health. It is critical to acknowledge that mental & physical health are equally significant & should be approached with the same consideration, compassion, & understanding. We can lessen stigma & establish a culture that values mental wellness by promoting an open & accepting atmosphere where people feel comfortable talking about their mental health. By incorporating mental health education, offering resources, & creating support networks for individuals in need, communities, workplaces, & schools can all play a significant role in fostering mental wellness. Other elements like emotional intelligence, self-worth, & social support are also strongly associated with mental wellness. The ability to recognise, comprehend, & control one's own emotions as well as those of others is known as emotional intelligence, & it is crucial for preserving mental health. People with high emotional intelligence are typically better at handling stress, forming enduring bonds with others, & settling disputes amicably. Emotional intelligence enables people to deal with challenging emotions, such as fear, sadness, or anger, without letting them control their actions. Mental wellness can also be significantly impacted by developing a positive sense of self-worth that is founded on acceptance of oneself rather than approval from others. People are more resilient in the face of adversity & are less likely to give in to feelings of anxiety, depression, or self-doubt when they are confident in themselves & feel good about themselves. Another important element that affects mental wellness is social support. Strong bonds with friends, family, or other neighbours give people a feeling of emotional stability, belonging, & connection. During trying times, having a support system can provide a safety net by allowing people to talk about their difficulties, get support, & feel understood. Since people who feel supported are typically better able to handle hardship & recover from setbacks, social support can also serve as a stress-reduction strategy. Additionally, work-life balance—which is becoming more & more crucial in today's fast-paced, constantly-connected world—is closely related to mental wellness. Burnout, stress, & a feeling of overwhelm are frequently caused by the demands of both work & personal life. Maintaining mental wellness requires striking a work-life balance because it enables people to schedule downtime for social interaction, self-care, & relaxation. Preventing burnout & promoting mental health require establishing clear boundaries between work & personal life, setting reasonable expectations, & making time for relaxation & leisure activities a priority. It's critical to keep in mind that mental wellness is an ongoing process rather than a final destination. Maintaining it calls for constant focus, self-awareness, & work, particularly when dealing with life's unavoidable ups & downs. Being mentally healthy is a dynamic & ever-changing process, & navigating life's ups & downs requires self-compassion & patience. People can develop resilience, enhance their quality of life, & create long-lasting mental well-being by implementing mental wellness-promoting behaviours into their daily routines, getting help when necessary, & creating a supportive environment. In the end, making an investment in mental wellness is an investment in relationships, productivity, general happiness, & physical health. Like physical health, it is a fundamental component of holistic health & should be given the same priority & care. A dedication to mental health enables people to not only manage but also flourish in the face of life's obstacles.

Stress & Its Connection To Cancer

Because of its extensive effects on both physical & mental health, stress in all of its manifestations has long been a topic of interest & concern in the medical & psychological domains. The link between stress & cancer is among the most fascinating & intricate relationships that researchers have looked into. Although stress does not directly cause cancer, an increasing amount of scientific research indicates that long-term or chronic stress may have a substantial impact on the onset & spread of cancer by altering a number of bodily biological processes. Investigating the physiological processes that support the body's stress response & how they might interact with cellular growth, mutation, & immune system function—all of which are important elements in the development of cancer—is necessary to comprehend this connection. The sympathetic nervous system is activated during the body's natural stress response, also known as the "fight or flight" response, which results in the release of hormones like cortisol & adrenaline. These hormones are generally beneficial in small amounts & during brief periods of stress because they prime the body to react rapidly to perceived dangers. The continuous release of these hormones, however, can impair the body's capacity to operate at its best when stress becomes chronic or ongoing, particularly with regard to the immune system, inflammation, & cellular integrity. The immune system is one of the main ways that long-term stress can affect the development of cancer. To detect & remove aberrant cells from the body, including cancerous or precancerous cells, a robust immune system is necessary. Long-term stress, however, has been demonstrated to impair the immune system's capacity to identify & eliminate these cells. Immune system alterations brought on by stress can raise the risk of cancer by enabling aberrant cells to multiply & avoid detection. For instance, stress can lower the activity & production of immune cells that are essential for the body's defence against cancer, such as T lymphocytes & natural killer cells. Furthermore, stress can encourage the body's inflammatory response, which is known to accelerate the development of cancer. Pro-inflammatory cytokines & other chemicals that can cause inflammation in different tissues have been connected to the release of chronic stress. Since inflammation can result in the formation of a microenvironment that promotes tumour growth, it is a known factor in the development & spread of cancer. Additionally, this inflammation may encourage cancer cells to spread (metastasise) to other areas of the body, making treatment & management of the disease more challenging. Stress may also contribute to cancer by indirectly raising a person's risk through behavioural changes. People who suffer from long-term stress, for instance, are more likely to use unhealthy coping strategies like smoking, binge drinking, eating poorly, & not exercising. It is well known that these lifestyle choices raise the chance of getting lung, liver, & colorectal cancer, among other cancers. Moreover, the relationship between stress & cancer encompasses not only the onset of the illness but also its advancement & reaction to therapy. According to research, people who are under a lot of stress are more likely to have worse outcomes—such as lower survival rates—after receiving a cancer diagnosis. By reducing immune function, changing hormone levels, & creating an environment that encourages tumour growth, stress can impair the body's capacity to fight cancer. Furthermore, stress can have an impact on a patient's compliance with cancer treatment because it can cause exhaustion, anxiety, depression, & trouble focussing, all of which can make it harder to adhere to treatment plans or keep a positive attitude. Feelings of helplessness, anxiety, & fear brought on by a cancer diagnosis & treatment can also add to the emotional toll of the illness, intensifying the stress response & possibly making the healing process more difficult. Changes in hormone levels are one of the biological pathways through which stress can impact cancer. Cortisol, sometimes known as the "stress hormone," is one of the most significant hormones in the stress response. In order to help the body deal with the perceived threat, the adrenal glands release cortisol when stress occurs. Cortisol affects the body in many ways, such as lowering inflammation, suppressing the immune system, & raising blood sugar. These effects aid the body's reaction to acute stress in the short term. However, the immune system is weakened & inflammation rises when cortisol levels stay high for long periods of time, which is frequently the case in chronic stress. These conditions can provide an environment that is conducive to the growth of cancer cells. Furthermore, it has been demonstrated that stress raises levels of other hormones like norepinephrine & adrenaline, which can encourage the growth of cancer cells & aid in the spread of tumours. For example, it has been discovered that adrenaline stimulates angiogenesis, the process by which blood vessels that supply tumours grow. Adrenaline speeds up the growth & spread of tumours by boosting their blood supply. Additionally, stress can change how cancer cells behave, making them more hostile & treatment-resistant. Studies have shown that stress hormones can affect cancer cells by encouraging apoptosis, the process by which cells avoid dying. Apoptosis typically occurs in damaged or aberrant cells to stop them from proliferating & developing into tumours. Stress hormones, however, have the ability to obstruct this process, enabling aberrant cells to endure & multiply. Stress can affect cancer risk not only directly through biological effects but also through behavioural pathways. Chronic stressors are more likely to participate in unhealthy behaviours that raise their risk of developing cancer, as was previously mentioned. Stress, for instance, may increase a person's propensity to smoke or drink alcohol, both of which are known to cause cancer. Stress can also result in unhealthy eating patterns, such as overindulging in unhealthy foods or skipping exercise, which raises the risk of obesity & some types of cancer. Sleep disturbances have also been connected to chronic stress, which can further impair the body's capacity to control inflammation & preserve a strong immune system. Numerous health problems, including an elevated risk of cancer, have been linked to inadequate sleep. Furthermore, the gut microbiota, which is becoming more widely acknowledged as a significant contributor to the development of cancer, can be impacted by stress. The trillions of bacteria, viruses, & fungi that live in the gastrointestinal tract & are essential to immunological response & general health make up the gut microbiome. Prolonged stress can change the gut microbiome's makeup, creating an imbalance of good & bad bacteria that may influence the development of cancer by altering inflammation & immune function. Although a lot has been discovered recently, there is still much to learn about the specific mechanisms through which stress affects cancer risk & progression. The relationship between stress & cancer is complex. It is evident, nevertheless, that stress management plays a significant role in the prevention & treatment of cancer in general. People can take proactive measures to lower stress & enhance mental wellness as part of a comprehensive approach to cancer prevention, given the possible role that stress may play in the development of cancer. Effective stress-reduction methods that can enhance mental & physical health include mindfulness, meditation, deep breathing exercises, & physical activities like yoga & exercise. Support from friends, family, or mental health specialists is also essential for assisting people in managing the psychological effects of stress & cancer. Reducing stress through therapy, lifestyle modifications, & other interventions may lower the risk of developing cancer & enhance the prognosis of individuals who have already been diagnosed. Although stress cannot always be prevented, there are significant advantages to learning how to effectively manage it for both cancer prevention & general health.

Mindfulness & Relaxation Techniques

Techniques for mindfulness & relaxation are crucial for stress management, enhancing mental clarity, & cultivating a more profound sense of wellbeing. People are realising more & more how important mindfulness & relaxation techniques are to preserving both physical & mental health in today's hectic & frequently overwhelming world. These methods, which include progressive muscle relaxation, body scan exercises, mindfulness meditation, deep breathing exercises, & guided imagery, provide a means of calming the mind, lowering anxiety, & developing present-focused awareness. Fundamentally, mindfulness is focussing entirely on the here & now without passing judgement.

Because it encourages people to observe their thoughts, emotions, & bodily sensations without becoming overwhelmed or reactive to them, this straightforward yet profound practice has the potential to change people's lives. Through mindfulness, people can overcome the mental clutter that frequently impairs their capacity to think clearly & feel at ease by learning to accept the present moment instead of becoming mired in a cycle of worry, rumination, or anxiety about the past or future. Studies have demonstrated that consistent mindfulness practice can result in long-lasting changes in brain structure & function, particularly in areas related to emotional regulation, self-awareness, & attention. These benefits of mindfulness go beyond mental clarity & stress reduction. The prefrontal cortex, a region of the brain involved in higher cognitive processes like attention, impulse control, & decision-making, has been shown to thicken as a result of mindfulness meditation. The hippocampus, which is essential for memory & emotional control, can also become more active as a result of mindfulness. The long-term mental health advantages of mindfulness, including enhanced resilience, elevated mood, & a better capacity to handle stress, are believed to be facilitated by these brain alterations. Regular mindfulness practice can also assist people in developing compassion, empathy, & thankfulness for others as well as for themselves. Mindfulness meditation is one of the most popular mindfulness techniques. It usually entails sitting comfortably, paying attention to the breath, & bringing the mind's focus back to the present moment whenever distractions occur. Focused attention meditation, open monitoring meditation, & loving-kindness meditation are just a few of the various types of mindfulness meditation that are based on the idea of non-judgmental awareness. Developing a sense of awareness & acceptance without attempting to alter or control the experience is the key to mindfulness meditation. In order to create a space for healing & self-discovery, mindfulness meditation encourages people to acknowledge unpleasant thoughts & feelings with curiosity & openness rather than repressing or avoiding them. An additional effective relaxation method that can aid in triggering the body's relaxation response is deep breathing exercises, which are frequently combined with mindfulness exercises. Our breath tends to become rapid & shallow when we are stressed or anxious, which can exacerbate tension & uneasiness. By encouraging slow, deep, & deliberate breaths, deep breathing techniques like diaphragmatic breathing, belly breathing, or the 4-7-8 technique help to counteract this stress response. The parasympathetic nervous system, which controls the body's "rest & digest" processes, is stimulated by these breathing techniques, which lowers blood pressure, heart rate, & promotes calmness & relaxation. Regular deep breathing exercises can also help people become more adept at handling stress in real time, which enables them to react to difficult circumstances with more composure & clarity. For instance, centring the mind & preventing overwhelming emotions from taking over can be achieved by taking a few deep breaths prior to a stressful meeting or presentation. Progressive muscle relaxation, or PMR, is another well-liked relaxation method that entails methodically tensing & relaxing various body muscle groups. By encouraging a stronger sense of connection between the mind & body, this technique assists people in becoming more conscious of the physical sensations of tension & relaxation. PMR helps lessen the physical signs of stress, like tightness in the jaw, shoulders, or lower back, by intentionally releasing muscle tension. Because it enables both mental & physical relaxation, PMR is especially beneficial for people who carry physical tension due to ongoing stress or anxiety. Another relaxation method is guided imagery, sometimes referred to as visualisation, which entails using the imagination to conjure up images of serene, tranquil, or upbeat situations. Because it enables people to withdraw from their immediate surroundings & enter a mental haven of peace, this practice can be particularly beneficial for lowering stress & anxiety. Although guided imagery can be performed independently, it is frequently more successful when facilitated by a qualified professional, such as a relaxation coach, therapist, or audio recording. People are urged to picture particular settings or scenes that arouse feelings of tranquilly, like a beach, a forest, or a mountaintop, during a guided imagery session. People can feel a deep sense of relaxation by mentally engrossing themselves in these uplifting pictures, which can lessen stress, anxiety, & elevate mood in general. It has been demonstrated that guided imagery is especially useful for lowering anxiety & depressive symptoms & enhancing the quality of sleep. Additionally, the practice facilitates mental clarity & relaxation by encouraging people to use their imagination & creativity. Another mindfulness-based method is body scan meditation, which entails methodically going over the entire body from head to toe, focussing on each area, & noting any places of stress, discomfort, or relaxation. People who engage in this practice gain a greater sense of body awareness & become more sensitive to their body's sensations. Because it encourages people to pay mindful attention to the parts of their bodies that require relaxation & care, the body scan is especially helpful for people who suffer from chronic physical tension or pain. Regular body scan practice helps people recognise & release tension before it becomes too much to handle, which helps them avoid stress & physical discomfort. Body scan meditation can also help people sleep better because it promotes calmness & relaxation, which makes it easier for people to fall asleep & stay asleep all night. The capacity of mindfulness & relaxation techniques to assist people in better emotional regulation is one of their main features. One of the most important components of mental wellness is emotional regulation, which is the capacity to control & react to emotional experiences in a healthy & adaptive manner. Mindfulness & relaxation techniques can assist people in recognising & accepting intense emotions, like sadness, anger, or frustration, without becoming overcome by them. By engaging in mindfulness practices, people can observe their feelings objectively & fully experience them without becoming overwhelmed by them. Instead of reacting rashly or letting their emotions rule them, this gives people the freedom to decide how they want to react to their emotions. Therefore, in the face of life's obstacles, mindfulness & relaxation techniques can assist people in developing healthier coping mechanisms, lowering emotional reactivity, & increasing emotional resilience. Regular mindfulness & relaxation exercises have been linked to long-term improvements in mental & physical health, according to research. Research shows that practicing mindfulness meditation or other relaxation methods can improve cognitive function, memory, & attention while lowering stress, anxiety, & depressive symptoms. By encouraging relaxation & lessening the damaging effects of stress on the body, these techniques have also been shown to lower the risk of developing chronic illnesses like diabetes, high blood pressure, & heart disease. Additionally, it has been demonstrated that mindfulness & relaxation practices strengthen the immune system, promote better sleep, & raise general feelings of wellbeing. These advantages highlight how crucial it is to integrate mindfulness & relaxation techniques into daily life since they can assist people in managing stress, enhancing their mental well-being, & improving their quality of life. To sum up, mindfulness & relaxation methods are effective means of enhancing both mental & physical health. People can lower stress, enhance emotional regulation, & develop a stronger sense of connection with themselves & the present moment by practicing mindfulness, deep breathing, progressive muscle relaxation, guided imagery, or body scan meditation. These behaviours are crucial parts of a healthy, balanced lifestyle because they can help people become more resilient, deal with difficulties more skilfully, & improve their general well-being. Including mindfulness & relaxation practices in daily routines can result in long-lasting gains in emotional stability, mental clarity, & physical health, giving people the skills they need to prosper in a world that is becoming more & more stressful.

Sleep: The Unsung Hero Of Cancer Prevention

In addition to its profound & frequently underappreciated role in preserving health, new research indicates that sleep is crucial for preventing cancer. Beyond just acknowledging the importance of getting enough sleep, the complex relationship between sleep & cancer includes knowing how different sleep stages affect immune system performance, DNA repair, hormone regulation, & the body's capacity to fend off the growth of cancerous cells. Sleep is an active process that influences many physiological functions necessary for preserving health, rather than just being a passive state of rest. As oxidative stress, inflammation, & cellular damage are all linked to the development & spread of cancer, sleep—especially deep & restorative sleep—is actually a critical time for the body to engage in repair & regeneration processes. As studies progress, researchers have found that sleep deprivation or disturbance can impair these vital body processes, increasing the likelihood that cancerous cells will develop, multiply, & avoid detection. We must investigate the biological processes by which sleep affects our immune system, genetic integrity, hormonal balance, & general cancer susceptibility in order to completely comprehend the significant impact of sleep on cancer prevention. The impact of sleep on immune function is among the most well-established links between sleep & cancer. In order to identify & eradicate aberrant cells—including cancerous ones—before they have an opportunity to proliferate & spread, the immune system is crucial. Rogue cells must be found & eliminated by the body's natural immune defences, which include specialised white blood cells like macrophages, cytotoxic T lymphocytes, & natural killer (NK) cells. However, sleep is the best time for this immune surveillance process, especially during deep sleep stages, also referred to as slow-wave sleep (SWS). The body produces more cytokines—proteins that control immune responses—during these stages, which strengthens the body's defences against infections & aberrant cell division. Additionally, it has been demonstrated that sleep has an impact on the generation of specific immune cells that are essential for the detection & destruction of cancerous cells. According to research, sleep deprivation—whether from poor sleep quality, insufficient sleep duration, or disrupted sleep patterns—can dramatically lower these immune cells' activity, impairing the body's defences &

raising the risk of developing cancer. Additionally, it has been demonstrated that getting too little sleep raises the synthesis of pro-inflammatory cytokines, which are linked to chronic low-grade inflammation—a condition known to play a significant role in the development & spread of cancer. Because it produces a microenvironment that can promote tumour growth, angiogenesis (the creation of new blood vessels to supply tumours), & metastasis (the spread of cancer cells to other parts of the body), inflammation plays a crucial role in the development of cancer. Furthermore, inflammation raises the risk of cancer by causing normal cells to undergo mutations & DNA damage. Therefore, insufficient sleep indirectly contributes to the conditions required for cancer development by increasing inflammation. DNA repair is another important sleep-related factor in cancer prevention. Sleep is essential for maintaining genetic integrity & repairing damaged cells. The body is subjected to a variety of environmental stressors throughout the day, such as pollutants, UV rays, & metabolic waste products that can harm DNA. The body goes through a restorative phase while we sleep, during which time DNA repair mechanisms are triggered to fix the damage & return the cells to normal function. The body uses sleep, especially the deep sleep & REM (rapid eye movement) phases, to repair DNA damage brought on by environmental factors & oxidative stress. When it comes to preventing mutations that may cause cancer, this restorative function is especially crucial. Conversely, long-term sleep deprivation impairs the body's capacity to correctly repair DNA, making cells more susceptible to genetic mutations that can cause cancer. Due to its detrimental effects on DNA repair processes, sleep deprivation has been associated with an increased risk of developing a number of cancers, including lung, colorectal, prostate, & breast cancer. Additionally, the circadian rhythm—the body's internal biological clock that controls the sleep-wake cycle—is crucial for preserving genetic stability. The body's capacity to repair DNA & control cell growth can be hampered by circadian rhythm disruptions, such as those brought on by shift work, jet lag, or irregular sleep patterns, which increases the risk of cancer. This link between DNA repair & sleep emphasises how crucial regular, high-quality sleep is for lowering the risk of cancer & preserving general health. Another important component of the link between sleep & cancer prevention is hormonal regulation. Sleep has a significant impact on the release of several hormones that are directly related to the risk of cancer, such as insulin, cortisol, & melatonin. The pineal gland releases melatonin, sometimes known as the "sleep hormone," in reaction to darkness. Melatonin is essential for controlling sleep cycles & preserving the circadian rhythm of the body. Melatonin has been demonstrated to have anti-cancer effects in addition to its ability to promote sleep. It is a potent antioxidant that shields cells from oxidative stress. It has also been shown to stop cancer cells from growing & slow the spread of tumours. Additionally, melatonin controls the synthesis of oestrogen, which has been linked to the emergence of some hormone-related cancers, including ovarian & breast cancer. Melatonin production can be decreased by chronic sleep disturbance or sleep deprivation, which raises the risk of hormone-related cancers. Conversely, getting enough sleep promotes optimal melatonin levels, which may offer some cancer prevention benefits. Another significant factor in the link between sleep & cancer is the stress hormone cortisol. In reaction to stress, the adrenal glands release cortisol, which aids in controlling a number of body processes such as inflammation, immunological response, & metabolism. In accordance with its natural circadian rhythm, cortisol peaks in the morning to aid in the body's awakening & progressively declines throughout the day. However, irregular or inadequate sleep can cause cortisol levels to become unbalanced, which can result in long-term increases in cortisol. This can raise inflammation, interfere with hormonal balance, & negatively impact immune function—all of which raise the risk of cancer. A vicious cycle that increases the risk of cancer is created by prolonged stress, inadequate sleep, & high cortisol levels. Finally, sleep affects weight regulation & metabolism, which in turn affects cancer prevention. Poor sleep has been linked to a higher risk of obesity, diabetes, & metabolic syndrome, all of which are risk factors for a number of cancer types, according to research. Lack of sleep alters how hunger hormones like ghrelin & leptin are regulated, which increases appetite & causes bad eating habits that can lead to weight gain & obesity. Because excess body fat can result in insulin resistance, hormonal imbalances, & chronic inflammation—all of which encourage the development of cancer—obesity is a known risk factor for a number of cancers, including colorectal, breast, & endometrial cancer. Lack of sleep has also been linked to increased insulin resistance & impaired glucose metabolism, both of which raise the risk of type 2 diabetes & cancer. Thus, keeping a healthy sleep schedule is crucial to preserving a healthy weight & lowering the risk of cancer. Sleep has a complex role in preventing cancer & is crucial for preserving general health & wellbeing. Sleep is essential for defending the body against the onset & spread of cancer because of its effects on metabolism, inflammation, immune system function, DNA repair, & hormone regulation. However, a lot of people in today's modern society experience poor sleep quality or sleep deprivation, which can be brought on by stress, lifestyle choices, or work schedules. Prioritising proper sleep hygiene & making sure the body gets the restorative sleep it requires each night are essential for lowering the risk of cancer & promoting general health. This entails keeping a regular sleep schedule, making the space conducive to rest, minimising screen time prior to bed, & using relaxation methods to reduce stress. In order to address these problems & enhance the quality of their sleep, people who suffer from sleep disorders like insomnia or sleep apnoea should also get medical help. People can take proactive measures to safeguard their health & lower their risk of developing cancer by being aware of & appreciating the significant influence that sleep has on cancer prevention. To sum up, sleep is an unsung hero in the fight against cancer, & its significance for preserving bodily health cannot be emphasised enough. A vital part of preventing cancer & maintaining general health is making sure the body gets enough good sleep every night. People's quality of life & cancer risk can be considerably decreased by making sleep a priority & forming healthy sleep habits.

Cultivating A Positive Outlook On Health

A vital but frequently disregarded component of wellbeing, maintaining a positive attitude towards one's health can have a significant impact on one's physical & mental health. It is more important than ever to cultivate a mindset that prioritises optimism, resilience, & proactive care in a world where stress, negativity, & chronic illness are prevalent experiences. A positive attitude towards health affects how people view their own health as well as how they behave, cope, & live their lives in general. The cultivation of optimism, gratitude, self-compassion, & a growth-oriented mindset are all components of the multifaceted idea of a positive outlook. People are more likely to adopt behaviours that promote their physical, mental, & emotional well-being when they cultivate & maintain a positive attitude towards their health. This entails adopting a healthier lifestyle, getting medical attention when needed, engaging in regular exercise, & effectively handling stress. Furthermore, people who have a positive attitude about their health also typically have lower levels of stress, anxiety, & depression—all of which are linked to a number of health problems, such as immunological dysfunction, cardiovascular disease, & chronic pain conditions. People can enhance their body's capacity to handle sickness, heal from wounds, & delay the onset of disease by cultivating an optimistic outlook. This way of thinking about health is based on the notion that mental & emotional states can directly affect physical health & that the mind & body are closely related. Positive attitudes have been linked to better health outcomes, adherence to medical advice, & preventative health behaviours, according to numerous studies. Numerous studies indicate that those who have a positive outlook on life are less likely to suffer from long-term illnesses like cancer, diabetes, & heart disease. This phenomenon, which is frequently called the "mind-body connection," emphasises how crucial mental health is in affecting physical health. Optimism, for instance, has been connected to better cardiovascular health, increased immunological response, & decreased inflammation. On the other hand, people who have pessimistic or negative outlooks might be more stressed & anxious, which can lead to high blood pressure, compromised immune systems, & a higher chance of chronic illnesses. There is strong scientific evidence to support the idea that our thoughts & emotions can affect our physical health; it is not just a theory. Positive thinking has a complex effect on health through a number of physiological pathways, such as the autonomic nervous system, immune system, & stress hormone regulation. The body is better able to control stress & inflammation, two factors that are connected to the emergence of chronic illnesses, when people have a positive outlook. Conversely, a pessimistic mindset frequently triggers the release of stress hormones like cortisol & adrenaline, which can weaken the immune system, raise blood pressure, & aid in the onset of illness. The practice of gratitude is one of the most crucial elements of developing a positive perspective on health. Numerous psychological & physical advantages of gratitude have been demonstrated, such as increased immunity, better sleep, & an overall sense of well-being. People can change their perspective from what is lacking or incorrect in their lives to what is abundant & positive by regularly practicing gratitude. This straightforward but effective technique can help people reframe unpleasant experiences & cultivate gratitude for the body's abilities & health. Regular gratitude practice has been linked to better mental health, increased life satisfaction, & even a decrease in the symptoms of chronic pain, according to research. In terms of health, this can entail focussing less on perceived flaws or limitations & more on the little everyday successes, like getting enough sleep, eating healthily, or exercising. People can strengthen their foundation of mental & emotional resilience, which in turn supports their physical health, by identifying & appreciating the positive aspects of health. Another essential element of developing a positive perspective on health is self-compassion. It entails showing oneself the same consideration, consideration, & kindness that one would show a close friend or loved one. When it comes to health, self-compassion encourages people to treat themselves with kindness during times of illness, setbacks, or health difficulties. Self-compassion focusses on acceptance & forgiveness rather than blaming oneself for perceived flaws or failures in one's health, enabling people to approach health with tolerance & understanding. Self-compassion has been demonstrated to improve emotional well-being, lessen the psychological toll of chronic illness, & improve overall health outcomes. People are more likely to adopt health-promoting behaviours & ask for assistance when needed when they practise self-compassion. Additionally, by lowering feelings of guilt, shame, or frustration that may surface when coping with health issues, self-compassion can promote a positive outlook. Self-compassion encourages people to see illness & health struggles as a natural part of life rather than as failures, which lessens the emotional distress that frequently accompanies health issues. Another essential component of a positive outlook on health is having a growth-oriented mindset, which views obstacles & failures as chances for development. Resilience & the capacity to adjust to shifting conditions rather than being overcome by them are highlighted by this way of thinking. When it comes to health, a growth mindset encourages people to view challenges like disease or injury as transient & controllable rather than insurmountable. People are more likely to look for answers, change their lifestyles, & take proactive measures to improve their health when they have a growth mindset. A person with a growth mindset, for example, might see a medical diagnosis as an opportunity to prioritise self-care, eat better, or exercise more. By encouraging a sense of empowerment rather than helplessness, this way of thinking can assist people in navigating the highs & lows of health with more ease & optimism. The importance of social support & connection is another essential component of developing a positive attitude towards health. Our relationships with others have a big impact on our physical & emotional well-being. In times of illness or health difficulties, supportive social networks—whether they be with family, friends, or support groups—can offer practical assistance, emotional support, & encouragement. Strong social ties have been linked in studies to longer lifespans, better immune systems, & lower rates of chronic illness. Additionally, social support can mitigate the detrimental impacts of stress & anxiety, two factors that can impede well-being & exacerbate illness. Positive relationships also support healthy habits like consistent exercise, a balanced diet, & stress reduction, all of which enhance general wellbeing. On the other hand, toxic or unfavourable relationships can be harmful to one's health, increasing stress, emotional distress, & the likelihood of mental health problems. Therefore, developing a positive outlook on health requires cultivating positive relationships & surrounding oneself with supportive people. Setting reasonable expectations & goals is another crucial factor to take into account when developing a positive attitude towards health. It is critical to recognise that maintaining good health is a lifelong process that calls for self-control, consistent effort, & reasonable expectations. People can increase their confidence in their capacity to preserve & enhance their health by establishing attainable health goals & acknowledging minor victories. Setting small, achievable goals, like walking more each day, getting better sleep, or eating more fruits & vegetables, gives people a sense of accomplishment & motivation, which in turn promotes optimism. Conversely, unrealistic expectations can undermine one's health efforts & general well-being by causing frustration, disappointment, & feelings of failure. Therefore, developing a long-lasting positive outlook on health requires setting reasonable goals that are in line with one's abilities & lifestyle. Developing a positive mindset can also be achieved by integrating mindfulness into one's approach to health. Applying mindfulness to different facets of health, such as stress management, exercise, & food, entails focussing on the here & now without passing judgement. People who are aware of their bodies' needs are better able to make health-related decisions, such as eating wholesome foods, exercising, & using healthy coping mechanisms for stress. Additionally, mindfulness fosters a greater appreciation for one's body & its potential, which improves one's sense of wellbeing in general. Furthermore, mindfulness promotes accepting one's body as it is rather than aiming for impractical goals or evaluating oneself against others. Long-term health & well-being depend on having a positive relationship with one's body & health, which is fostered by this acceptance. Lastly, it's critical to understand that developing a positive perspective on health is an ongoing process rather than an isolated incident. It takes constant work, introspection, & self-care to keep a positive attitude in the face of life's obstacles, disappointments, & unexpected turns. Through regular mindfulness, self-compassion, resilience, & gratitude exercises, people can develop a mindset that promotes their health & wellbeing. Furthermore, adopting a positive perspective on health involves embracing the entire range of health, including mental, physical, emotional, & spiritual, rather than merely emphasising the absence of disease. People can lower their chance of developing chronic diseases, increase their capacity to handle stress & adversity, & improve their general quality of life by adopting a positive outlook & a holistic approach to health. To sum up, developing a positive perspective on health is a potent & life-changing technique that can raise general wellbeing & enhance health results. People can develop a stronger bond with their bodies, make better decisions, & lower their risk of illness by adopting an optimistic, resilient, & proactive mindset. By practicing mindfulness, self-compassion, growth-oriented thinking, gratitude, & social support, people can build a foundation of mental & emotional resilience that promotes their health & gives them the ability to lead active, satisfying lives.

Building Resilience Through Mental Wellness

A key strategy for overcoming life's obstacles is developing resilience via mental wellness, especially in the modern world where stress, uncertainty, & misfortune are frequent occurrences. The capacity to bounce back from setbacks, adjust to adversity, & preserve mental & emotional health in the face of hardship is resilience. It entails developing a mindset that prioritises optimism, tenacity, & the possibility of progress in addition to managing stress & becoming stronger as a result. The development of emotional intelligence—the capacity to identify, comprehend, & effectively regulate one's emotions as well as to empathise with others—is one of the most important components of resilience building. Emotional intelligence reduces impulsive reactions & promotes healthier, more constructive responses to challenges by assisting people in responding to life's challenges in a thoughtful & balanced way. Additionally, it is crucial for improving relationships, communication, & problem-solving skills—all of which are critical components of resilience. Maintaining mental wellness requires emotional regulation, which is a facet of emotional intelligence. How well a person handles adversity can be determined by their capacity to regulate & control their emotional reactions, whether they are to stress, frustration, or disappointment. Techniques like deep breathing, mindfulness, & meditation are useful for developing emotional regulation because they keep people rooted in the here & now & lessen the impact of negative emotions. These methods also help people become more self-aware, which is essential for recognising their emotional triggers & learning how to react in ways that are more consistent with their values

& objectives. Positive thinking & cognitive reframing—which entails altering how one perceives & reacts to adverse events—further enhance resilience. People are better able to cope with adversity when they see challenges as chances for growth & learning rather than insurmountable barriers. Optimism, which has been demonstrated to have several positive effects on both mental & physical health, such as lowering the risk of depression, boosting coping skills, & strengthening the immune system, is fostered by positive thinking. Cognitive reframing is a technique that helps people confront negative thought patterns & swap them out for more empowering, balanced viewpoints. The development of a growth mindset—a theory put forth by psychologist Carol Dweck—is a crucial component of resilience building. It entails the conviction that aptitude & intelligence can be enhanced via hard work, education, & persistence. By motivating people to see difficulties as chances to learn new skills, get past barriers, & become stronger, a growth mindset promotes resilience. On the other hand, a fixed mindset, in which people think their skills are unalterable & unchanging, can make them feel defeated & powerless when faced with challenges. Adopting a growth mindset supports people in preserving their sense of agency, control, & hope—all of which are critical elements of resilience. The formation of solid social ties is a key component in resilience building. Strong social support networks help people manage stress, heal from trauma, & preserve their mental health, according to numerous studies. In times of hardship, relationships with family, friends, & the community offer consolation, emotional support, & useful help. Social support fosters feelings of safety, belonging, & self-worth while acting as a buffer against the detrimental effects of stress. When faced with challenging situations, it also helps people keep perspective & serves as a source of inspiration, support, & direction. But it's crucial to understand that relationships' quality is more significant than their quantity. It is frequently better to have a small number of close, encouraging relationships rather than a large number of shallow ones. These solid bonds promote empathy, trust, & support for one another—all of which help people become more resilient. Furthermore, obtaining expert assistance, like counselling or therapy, can be an essential part of developing resilience. Professionals in mental health can offer helpful resources, coping mechanisms, & emotional support to help people get through challenging times & gradually increase their resilience. Another crucial characteristic of resilient people is psychological flexibility, or the capacity to adjust to shifting conditions & react nimbly to difficulties. Individuals with psychological flexibility can make deliberate decisions about how to handle hardship because they can accept their thoughts & feelings without being overcome by them. Because of this flexibility, people can modify their coping mechanisms as necessary, acknowledging that various circumstances may call for distinct methods. Building psychological flexibility entails learning to let go of strict expectations & judgements as well as practicing acceptance, mindfulness, & self-compassion. Developing a feeling of meaning & purpose in life is one of the most effective strategies to increase resilience. A distinct sense of purpose gives people focus, inspiration, & a reason to keep going when faced with obstacles in life. Even in the face of hardship, it helps people maintain their focus on their priorities. Strong senses of purpose have been linked to reduced stress, increased life satisfaction, & better health outcomes, according to research. Relationships, a job, hobbies, spiritual activities, or personal objectives are just a few of the many things that can give one a sense of purpose. Resilience is strengthened & a sense of fulfilment is fostered when one participates in activities that are consistent with their values & passions. Additionally, having a sense of purpose enables people to interpret challenging situations by seeing them as a necessary component of a broader path or process of personal development. This way of thinking can lessen hopelessness, encourage people to keep going despite obstacles, & lessen feelings of helplessness. Resilience & mental wellness are closely related to physical health. People who maintain their physical health through consistent exercise, a healthy diet, & enough sleep are better equipped to handle life's obstacles. Particularly, exercise has been demonstrated to lower stress, elevate mood, & improve cognitive function—all of which help people become more resilient. In addition to encouraging the growth of new brain cells, which improves emotional regulation & cognitive flexibility, physical activity increases the production of endorphins, which are naturally occurring mood enhancers. Exercise also enhances the quality of sleep, which is important for resilience & mental health. In order to ensure that people are physically capable of managing stress, proper nutrition promotes immune system health, mood regulation, & brain function. Because it enables the brain to process emotions & solidify memories from the day, getting enough sleep is crucial for emotional regulation, cognitive function, & general health. People who put their physical health first are more resilient because they can handle stress & bounce back from hardships more easily. Another essential element of developing resilience is self-care. To sustain mental wellness & build resilience, one must make time for both physical & emotional self-care. Self-care can include a variety of activities, including relaxation exercises, fun pursuits, boundary-setting, & putting one's own health first. Regular self-care enables people to rejuvenate, avoid burnout, & preserve a healthy outlook on life. Additionally, it fosters self-compassion & self-awareness, both of which are critical for developing a resilient mindset. Self-care is essential for developing resilience because it helps people refuel their physical & emotional reserves, giving them the fortitude to face obstacles head-on. By encouraging awareness, presence, & acceptance, mindfulness exercises can support people in developing resilience in addition to self-care. By concentrating on the here & now without passing judgement, mindfulness enables people to openly & curiously examine their thoughts, feelings, & bodily experiences. People can become more resilient, manage their emotions better, & experience less stress by practicing mindfulness. People can develop a sense of peace, clarity, & connection through mindfulness exercises like meditation, deep breathing, & mindful movement, which improves their capacity to handle hardship. Additionally, mindfulness makes people more conscious of their inner experiences, which empowers them to identify & question harmful thought patterns & beliefs. Additionally, gratitude fosters resilience. The practice of acknowledging & valuing life's good things, even when faced with difficulties, is known as gratitude. According to research, practicing gratitude can improve resilience overall, lower stress levels, & improve mental health. People's focus is diverted from negative thoughts & anxieties when they concentrate on their blessings, which promotes positivity & a sense of abundance. Additionally, gratitude enables people to reinterpret challenges as chances for development & education. Regular gratitude practice helps people become more resilient mentally & emotionally, which improves their capacity to handle life's obstacles. The capacity to accept & grow from failure is one of the main advantages of developing resilience via mental wellness. Resilient people see failure as a normal aspect of growth rather than a reflection of their value or skills. They recognise that failures & errors are not causes for self-doubt or discouragement, but rather present chances for growth & learning. Accepting failure as a teaching opportunity helps people become more resilient by motivating them to keep going when things get tough & stick to their objectives. Because people are less likely to be extremely critical of themselves when things don't go as planned, it also fosters self-compassion. Lastly, developing resilience is a dynamic, continuous process that calls for constant work & introspection. People must continue to be adaptable, flexible, & proactive in order to develop resilience through mental wellness because life is full of unknowns & difficulties. It is a journey rather than a destination that entails accepting change, growing from mistakes, & taking action to support one's mental & emotional well-being. People can increase their ability to overcome hardship & prosper in the face of life's obstacles by developing resilience-building techniques such as self-compassion, social support, emotional intelligence, & positive thinking. Developing resilience via mental health is a crucial ability that helps people face life's challenges with more ease, optimism, & tenacity.

CHAPTER 4: UNDERSTANDING ENVIRONMENTAL & LIFESTYLE RISKS

Comprehending the intricate & interconnected elements that impact our health, especially in regards to preventing chronic illnesses & advancing general well-being, requires an understanding of environmental & lifestyle hazards. Numerous diseases, such as respiratory disorders, cardiovascular disease, cancer, & neurological conditions, are frequently linked to environmental factors, which have a substantial impact on public health. These factors include air quality, water contamination, exposure to hazardous substances, & climate change. A person's physical, mental, & overall quality of life are all influenced by the surroundings in which they live, work, & interact. On the other hand, a person's risk for chronic diseases like diabetes, obesity, hypertension, & heart disease is greatly influenced by their lifestyle choices, which include things like food, exercise, smoking, alcohol use, sleep habits, & stress management. Since these lifestyle decisions are frequently changeable, people can drastically lower their chance of contracting these illnesses & enhance their long-term health results. However, lifestyle & environmental risks frequently coexist & have an impact on one another that can exacerbate their detrimental health effects. For instance, residing in an area with high air pollution levels can raise a person's risk of developing respiratory disorders, which can be made worse by smoking or leading a sedentary lifestyle.

In a similar vein, a poor diet & insufficient exercise can raise the risk of developing diseases like stroke, cancer, & type 2 diabetes in addition to obesity & metabolic disorders. People can take proactive measures to reduce environmental & lifestyle risks by being aware of the complex relationship between them. These measures may include changing one's lifestyle, advocating for environmental causes, or implementing preventive healthcare procedures. The different environmental & lifestyle risks, their role in disease, & methods to lessen their negative effects on health will all be covered in this chapter. Air pollution exposure is one of the main environmental health risks. Long-term exposure to pollutants like particulate matter (PM), nitrogen dioxide (NO2), sulphur dioxide (SO2), & ozone (O3) can raise the risk of respiratory conditions like asthma, chronic obstructive pulmonary disease (COPD), & lung cancer. Air quality is a significant determinant of respiratory health. Additionally, research has linked poor air quality to early mortality, stroke, & cardiovascular disease. The World Health Organisation (WHO) estimates that air pollution causes millions of deaths annually throughout the world, many of which are connected to prolonged exposure to contaminated air. There are serious health risks associated with both indoor & outdoor air pollution, & those who reside in cities with heavy traffic or industrial activity are especially at risk. Particularly for young children & the elderly, indoor air pollution—which is frequently brought on by tobacco smoke, cooking with solid fuels, & the use of specific household products—can also negatively impact respiratory health. In addition to respiratory problems, poor air quality can lead to mental health conditions like anxiety & depression & impair cognitive function. By avoiding outdoor exercise in busy places, using air purifiers indoors, & supporting laws that address environmental pollution—such as stronger emissions regulations & more green space in cities—people can lessen their exposure to air pollution. Water contamination, which can be brought on by sewage, industrial waste, agricultural runoff, & other pollutants getting into water sources, is another serious environmental risk. When ingested, contaminants like lead, arsenic, pesticides, & bacteria can have serious negative effects on health, especially for vulnerable groups like children, pregnant women, & the elderly. Developmental problems, neurological impairment, gastrointestinal disorders, & an elevated risk of some types of cancer can result from exposure to tainted water. The Flint water crisis in Michigan, where lead contamination in the drinking water caused numerous health issues & long-term developmental effects for children, is among the most well-known instances of water contamination. Furthermore, water scarcity & clean water availability are being made worse by climate change, especially in areas where droughts & other extreme weather events are occurring more frequently. Drinking filtered water, supporting laws that control water quality, & pushing for upgrades to water infrastructure can all help people lower their risk of drinking contaminated water. In addition to the quality of the air & water, exposure to dangerous chemicals &

environmental pollutants presents a serious health risk. Through food, water, air, & skin contact, industrial chemicals, pesticides, heavy metals, & endocrine-disrupting substances like phthalates & bisphenol A (BPA) can enter the body & cause a variety of health issues, such as hormone imbalances, cancers, reproductive disorders, & developmental delays. Another serious problem is occupational exposure to harmful chemicals like vinyl chloride, benzene, & asbestos. People who work in manufacturing, construction, & agriculture, for example, may be more susceptible to illness as a result of extended exposure. Using natural & non-toxic household products, adhering to safety procedures at work, & supporting laws that control the use of hazardous materials can all help reduce exposure to dangerous chemicals. Choosing organic food, safer personal care products, & non-toxic cleaning supplies are further ways that people can lessen their own exposure to chemicals. When it comes to disease prevention, lifestyle risks are equally important to take into account, & many of these risks are influenced by individual choices & habits. One important lifestyle factor that has a big impact on general health is diet. Obesity, diabetes, heart disease, & various cancers can be caused by a poor diet, which is defined by an excessive intake of processed foods, added sugars, unhealthy fats, & a deficiency of fruits, vegetables, & whole grains. Because of its high intake of trans fats, refined carbohydrates, & red & processed meats, the Western diet—often referred to as the "standard American diet"—is especially linked to an increased risk of developing chronic illnesses. On the other hand, a nutritious diet that prioritises whole, nutrient-dense foods like fruits, vegetables, lean meats, & whole grains can lower the risk of developing chronic illnesses & enhance general health. It has been demonstrated that the Mediterranean diet, which is high in plant-based foods, antioxidants, & healthy fats, reduces the risk of cancer, heart disease, & stroke. By eating a balanced, whole-foods-based diet & consuming fewer processed foods & sugary drinks, people can lower their risk of developing diet-related illnesses. Another essential lifestyle component for preserving health & lowering the risk of disease is regular physical activity. A major risk factor for diseases like obesity, heart disease, diabetes, & some types of cancer is sedentary behaviour, which is defined as extended periods of sitting or inactivity. Regular exercise, such as aerobic, strength, & flexibility training, can lower the risk of chronic diseases, improve mental health, control blood sugar, & improve cardiovascular health. To stay healthy, adults should engage in moderate-intensity exercise for at least 150 minutes each week, according to the American Heart Association. Additionally, physical activity can improve mood, improve cognitive function, & lessen the symptoms of anxiety & depression. People who exercise regularly are generally less likely to suffer from mental health issues & are more resilient to stress. The risk of disease is greatly increased by lifestyle factors like smoking & alcohol use in addition to diet & exercise. Smoking is linked to a number of cancers, especially lung cancer, as well as respiratory & cardiovascular conditions, making it one of the leading preventable causes of death. For nonsmokers, secondhand smoke exposure poses a serious health risk as well. One of the best strategies to lower the risk of these illnesses is to stop smoking or never start. Likewise, excessive alcohol use is associated with a number of cancers, heart issues, & liver disease. To lower the risk of alcohol-related health issues, the Centres for Disease Control & Prevention (CDC) advises people to limit their alcohol intake to no more than one drink for women & two for men per day. Additionally, sleep habits are essential for maintaining general health & preventing illness. Long-term sleep deprivation has been associated with a higher risk of heart disease, stroke, diabetes, obesity, & mental health issues. Immune system performance, memory consolidation, emotional control, & the body's capacity for self-repair & renewal all depend on sleep. For optimum health, adults should strive for 7-9 hours of sleep every night. The quality & length of sleep can be enhanced by adopting good sleep hygiene habits, such as sticking to a regular sleep schedule, developing a calming nighttime ritual, & reducing screen time before bed. Lastly, stress management is a critical component of both physical & mental health. Numerous health issues, such as heart disease, high blood pressure, digestive problems, & mental health disorders, are linked to chronic stress. The detrimental effects of stress on the body & mind can be lessened with the use of effective stress management strategies like deep breathing, mindfulness, meditation, & physical exercise. Including stress-reduction techniques in daily life can boost general wellbeing, increase resilience, & reduce the risk of diseases linked to stress. People can take charge of their health & enhance their quality of life by being aware of the lifestyle & environmental factors that increase the risk of disease & implementing preventative measures. In conclusion, a person's health outcomes are greatly influenced by both lifestyle & environmental factors. A poor diet, inactivity, smoking, excessive alcohol use, & exposure to air & water pollution, dangerous chemicals, & environmental pollutants can all have long-term health effects. People can greatly lower their risk of developing chronic diseases & improve their general well-being by making deliberate decisions to improve environmental conditions, limit exposure to dangerous substances, & adopt healthier lifestyle habits.

The Hidden Dangers Of Toxins In Daily Life

Even though toxins are present in our surroundings, homes, workplaces, & even the food we eat, their hidden risks in day-to-day living are frequently overlooked. These dangerous chemicals are present in commonplace materials & products, such as cleaning supplies, toiletries, food packaging, & even the air we breathe. Over time, toxins like heavy metals, pesticides, endocrine-disrupting chemicals, & volatile organic compounds (VOCs) can subtly enter our bodies & cause a variety of major health problems, from neurological disorders, reproductive issues, & developmental delays in children to chronic diseases like diabetes, cancer, &

heart disease. Because of a lack of awareness, a lack of regulation, or the fact that the substances are inconspicuous, the presence of these toxins in products that appear to be harmless can frequently go unnoticed. For instance, a lot of household cleaning products contain chemicals that release volatile organic compounds (VOCs), which can cause long-term lung damage, headaches, & respiratory problems when inhaled. Shampoos, lotions, & deodorants are examples of personal care products that may contain parabens, phthalates, & other endocrine-disrupting chemicals. These substances can disrupt the body's hormone balance & cause problems with reproduction & development. These chemicals can build up in the body through a process called bioaccumulation, which can result in long-term exposure & has been connected to a higher risk of developing certain cancers, birth defects, & other severe illnesses. Additionally, toxins are frequently found in food in the form of pesticides, food additives, artificial preservatives, & contaminants like heavy metals that can enter the food chain through environmental pollution or industrial processes. Fruits & vegetables absorb pesticides used in conventional farming, & some fish species can accumulate high levels of mercury & other toxins, which can be extremely harmful to human & environmental health. The air we breathe can contain invisible pollutants that can have long-term health effects, in addition to the toxins present in products. Fine particulate matter, nitrogen dioxide, sulphur dioxide, & other dangerous chemicals are found in both indoor & outdoor air pollution. These pollutants can harm the respiratory system, raise the risk of cardiovascular disease, & raise the chance of developing chronic illnesses like asthma, COPD, & even cancer. Exposure to these toxins puts the most vulnerable groups—children, the elderly, & people with underlying medical conditions—at heightened risk. Furthermore, because many chemicals do not have immediate, visible symptoms or immediate health consequences, toxins in daily life can frequently go unnoticed by conventional means. Exposure to these toxins can have long-term effects that build up over time, causing a silent health burden that may not be recognised until later in life when serious health conditions appear. The risk is that many people might not be aware of the possible risks associated with commonplace items & substances, which could result in continuous exposure that raises the risk over time. The fact that many common toxins are not subject to strict regulations, despite growing evidence of their detrimental effects, exacerbates the problem. The most recent scientific discoveries may not always be reflected in government regulations, exposing consumers to dangerous chemicals. In certain instances, industries prioritise profit over public health by lobbying to postpone or stop the implementation of safety standards. Since many companies are not required to disclose the complete list of ingredients or chemicals used in their products, this lack of regulatory oversight can leave people to fend for themselves when it comes to identifying & avoiding toxic substances. Bisphenol A (BPA), a chemical used in the production of plastic that has been connected to hormone disruption & an increased risk of cancer, is one example of a chemical that can seep into the food & beverages that are contained in seemingly innocuous products like food packaging. The endocrine system, which controls vital biological processes like metabolism, growth, & reproduction, is upset by many of these substances because they mimic hormones in the body. Plastic containers, cosmetics, cleaning supplies, & even toys are among the many consumer products that contain endocrine-disrupting chemicals (EDCs). Infertility, early puberty, & an elevated risk of hormone-related cancers like breast & prostate cancer are just a few of the health issues that can result from these chemicals' interference with hormone function once they are absorbed into the body. Lack of knowledge or comprehension of the cumulative effects of toxin exposure is one of the most alarming aspects of the situation. It's possible that many people are ignorant of the risks posed by everyday pollutants & fail to take precautions against their exposure. Furthermore, a lot of toxin-related health problems, like chronic diseases, neurological impairment, & hormonal imbalances, can appear gradually over time, making it challenging to pinpoint a specific toxin as the cause of their onset. Efforts to limit exposure may be made more difficult by the delayed onset of health effects, which can make it difficult for people to link their exposure to harmful substances to the emergence of health issues. Confusion is further increased by the rise in "greenwashing," the practice of businesses marketing goods as non-toxic or ecologically friendly without offering strong proof of their safety. Claims that products are free of hazardous chemicals frequently deceive consumers, who later learn that the products still contain potentially harmful substances. The frequency of toxic exposure in day-to-day activities emphasises the significance of taking preventative measures to reduce exposure & raise awareness. Making educated decisions about the products we use in our daily routines, workplaces, & homes is one of the best strategies to lower the risk of toxin exposure. The burden of toxins on the body can be considerably decreased, for example, by selecting organic or sustainably grown food, non-toxic cleaning products, & personal care products devoid of dangerous chemicals. Reducing exposure to potentially hazardous chemicals can also be achieved by choosing natural fibres for furniture & clothing, using non-toxic paints, & storing food in glass, stainless steel, or BPA-free plastic. To reduce exposure to dangerous substances at work, people can use personal protective equipment, promote improved safety procedures, & make sure there is enough ventilation. Public health protection at the societal level requires advocating for stricter laws & safety requirements for chemicals & poisons in consumer goods. Customers can also lend their support to environmental groups that strive to increase public awareness of the risks posed by toxins & push for legislative changes that would limit the use of dangerous chemicals. Addressing the hidden risks of toxins requires education & awareness because people need to know how to make safer decisions & what the long-term effects of exposure are. There are actions people can take to lessen their exposure, safeguard their health, & help create a safer, more sustainable environment for coming generations, even though completely removing all toxins from daily life may not be feasible. People can lower their risk of developing chronic illnesses & enhance their quality of life by taking proactive steps to limit their exposure to toxins. In the end, combating the hidden risks of toxins necessitates an all-encompassing strategy that incorporates increased public awareness, regulatory reform, & individual accountability. To create a healthier, toxin-free environment where people can flourish without worrying about hidden hazards in commonplace items & surroundings, governments, businesses, & individuals must work together.

The Role Of Smoking & Alcohol In Cancer Risk

It is impossible to overestimate the part that smoking & drinking alcohol play in the development of different types of cancer. These two lifestyle choices are among the most well-established & important ones that raise the risk of developing cancer. When taken separately or in combination, these drugs dramatically increase the risk of developing a number of cancers, such as breast, colorectal, liver, throat, & lung cancer for example. Smoking is the world's leading preventable cause of death, & studies have repeatedly shown a direct & unmistakable link between smoking & cancer. Since tobacco smoke contains over 7,000 chemicals, many of which are known to cause DNA mutations & the development of cancerous cells, its carcinogenic effects are well established. Benzene, formaldehyde, nitrosamines, & polycyclic aromatic hydrocarbons (PAHs) are the most powerful carcinogens found in tobacco smoke. These substances weaken the body's innate capacity to repair genetic damage, harm cellular structures, & encourage aberrant cell proliferation. Lung cancer is still the most common cause of cancer-related deaths globally, & cigarette smoking is especially well-known for its contribution to this disease. Compared to non-smokers, smokers have a 15–30 times higher risk of developing lung cancer. But the dangers are not limited to lung cancer; smoking is also closely associated with some forms of leukaemia & cancers of the mouth, throat, oesophagus, pancreas, bladder, kidney, stomach, & cervix. Both the length of time & the quantity of cigarettes smoked raise the risk of cancer, with those who have smoked for decades showing the highest risks. Secondhand smoke is a serious health risk to nonsmokers in addition to the direct carcinogenic effects of smoking, especially in enclosed areas where the harmful chemicals in tobacco smoke can build up & be inhaled. In the United States alone, secondhand smoke exposure is thought to be the cause of 41,000 deaths per year, many of which are attributable to heart disease & lung cancer. Since alcohol has been definitively associated with an increased risk of a number of cancers, including those of the mouth, throat, oesophagus, liver, colon, rectum, &

breast, the relationship between alcohol consumption & cancer risk is equally concerning. The main component of alcoholic beverages, ethanol, is broken down in the liver to produce the toxic & cancer-causing chemical acetaldehyde. Acetaldehyde raises the risk of cancer by damaging DNA, preventing the repair of genetic mutations, & encouraging aberrant cell division. Furthermore, drinking alcohol may hinder the body's absorption of vital nutrients, like folate, which are required for healthy DNA repair & cancer prevention. A person's risk of developing cancer is dose-dependent, meaning that the more alcohol they drink, the higher their risk. Particularly in women, even moderate drinking has been associated with an elevated risk of breast cancer. Because alcohol can raise the body's levels of oestrogen, studies have demonstrated a clear link between alcohol consumption & the development of oestrogen receptor-positive breast cancer, with the risk rising with each additional drink consumed daily. People with underlying liver diseases like cirrhosis or hepatitis & chronic alcohol use are at a higher risk of developing other cancers, like liver cancer. The risk of getting cancer is further increased by smoking & drinking alcohol, as these two behaviours work together to raise the risk of cancer development. This is particularly true for cancers of the mouth, throat, & oesophagus, where the combined risk of smoking & alcohol is much higher than that of either substance alone. According to research, people who smoke & drink together have a much higher chance of getting these cancers than people who just smoke or drink. Alcohol &

smoking are thought to have a synergistic effect on cancer risk because of their interactions with cells in the digestive & upper respiratory systems, which weaken the body's defences against the growth of cancerous cells & cause more DNA damage. The type of alcohol consumed also affects the risk of cancer; studies show that wine, spirits, & beer all raise the risk of cancer, though the exact risk may vary depending on the type of alcohol. Both alcohol & smoking have direct carcinogenic effects, but they can also raise the risk of cancer by fostering other illnesses that make people more vulnerable to the disease. For example, smoking increases the risk of developing chronic obstructive pulmonary disease (COPD), which impairs immunity & the lungs, leaving people more vulnerable to infections & cancer. However, alcohol can also lead to immune system suppression & liver disease, both of which increase the body's susceptibility to cancer. In addition to their direct effects on the development of cancer, smoking & drinking alcohol also raise the risk of developing cancer by contributing to poor general health. Heavy drinkers & smokers are more likely to partake in other unhealthy habits, like eating poorly & not exercising, which can also raise their risk of developing cancer. Furthermore, drinking & smoking can make other long-term health issues like diabetes & hypertension worse, which can raise the risk of cancer. Many people still smoke & drink alcohol in spite of the overwhelming evidence that these behaviours increase the risk of cancer. This is frequently because of addiction, social pressures, or a lack of knowledge about the risks involved. Because nicotine causes dopamine to be released in the brain, which results in pleasurable feelings & reinforces the behaviour, smoking is especially addictive. Although it can be challenging, quitting smoking is one of the best strategies to lower your risk of developing cancer & other smoking-related illnesses. After stopping smoking, the chance of getting cancer gradually declines; after only a few years of abstinence, former smokers' risk of getting cancer is significantly reduced. Alcohol can also become habitual, & people who drink too much may find it difficult to cut back or stop. This is because alcohol is not as physically addictive as smoking. Limiting alcohol intake, however, can dramatically reduce the risk of cancer, especially liver, breast, & digestive system cancers. Both alcohol & smoking are behaviours that people can control, & choosing to cut back or stop using either can significantly lower the risk of cancer & enhance general health. Cancer incidence can be significantly decreased by public health programs that support quitting smoking, increase knowledge of the dangers of alcohol, & promote healthier lifestyles. These programs may consist of educational campaigns, support groups, & tools for people who want to cut back on alcohol or stop smoking. The incidence of smoking & alcohol-related cancers can also be decreased by laws that control the marketing of tobacco & alcohol products, raise taxes on them, & limit their accessibility. Finally, the connection between alcohol & smoking & the risk of cancer emphasises how critical it is to make educated lifestyle decisions & take action to limit exposure to these carcinogens. Despite the fact that drinking alcohol & smoking are both deeply embedded in society & culture, people can lower their risk of developing cancer & make healthier decisions if they are aware of the major health risks connected to these behaviours. In addition to greatly reducing their risk of developing cancer, people can enhance their general health & quality of life by stopping smoking, drinking less alcohol, & looking for resources & support. The burden of smoking & alcohol-related cancers can be lessened, & a healthier, cancer-free future can be promoted, by society working together through education, policy changes, & support networks.

Protecting Your Skin From Uv Radiation

Maintaining skin health & avoiding a number of dangerous conditions, such as sunburn, skin cancer, & premature ageing, depend on protecting your skin from ultraviolet (UV) radiation. UV radiation is a type of electromagnetic radiation that can harm skin cells. It is mostly emitted by the sun, but it can also come from artificial sources like tanning beds. UVA & UVB are the two primary forms of UV radiation that have an impact on the skin. About 95% of UV radiation that reaches the Earth's surface is UVA radiation, which can penetrate the skin more deeply & cause long-term skin damage like wrinkles, age spots, & an elevated risk of skin cancer. Because UVB radiation mainly damages the epidermis, the skin's outermost layer, it is the cause of sunburn. Despite being less common than UVA radiation, UVB radiation is much more intense & is crucial in the development of skin cancers such as squamous cell carcinoma, basal cell carcinoma, & melanoma. UVA & UVB rays can both harm skin cells' DNA, causing mutations that build up over time & raise the risk of developing cancer. UV radiation has a well-established role in the development of skin cancer; research continuously demonstrates that individuals who are frequently sunburnt or who spend a lot of time in the sun without protection are much more likely to develop skin cancer in the future. Therefore, shielding the skin from UV rays is essential for lowering the risk of skin cancer & maintaining the general health of the skin. Using sunscreen is one of the best methods to shield the skin from UV rays. In order to stop UV rays from damaging the skin, sunscreen serves as a barrier. It's crucial to pick a sunscreen that offers broad-spectrum protection, which shields the skin from UVA & UVB rays. Additionally, the sunscreen should have a sun protection factor (SPF) of at least 30, meaning that 97% of UVB rays will be blocked by the product. A higher SPF of 50 or higher may offer extra protection for people with fair skin. All exposed skin, including frequently overlooked places like the ears, back of the neck, & tops of the feet, should have a thick layer of sunscreen applied. To guarantee ongoing protection, it's crucial to reapply sunscreen every two hours, or more frequently if you're swimming or perspiring. Wearing protective clothes is another efficient method of protecting the skin from UV rays, in addition to using sunscreen. High ultraviolet protection factor (UPF) clothing provides an additional line of defence against damaging UV radiation. An indicator of a fabric's ability to block UV rays is its UPF. A wide range of clothing items, such as hats, long-sleeved shirts, dresses, & trousers, are made of fabrics with a UPF of 50 or higher, which are thought to be very effective at blocking UV rays. Wearing a hat with a wide brim that protects the face, ears, & neck—areas of the body that are frequently exposed to the sun—is especially crucial. Furthermore, UV-blocking sunglasses can lower the risk of cataracts & other UV-related eye disorders while also protecting the sensitive skin around the eyes. In addition to wearing sunscreen & protective clothes, finding shade during the hottest parts of the day is another crucial measure in limiting UV exposure. Reducing sun exposure between 10 a.m. & 4 p.m., when the UV index is at its highest, is an efficient method of lowering the risk of skin damage because the sun's rays are at their strongest during this time. It's crucial to arrange outdoor activities in areas with shade, like beneath a tree, umbrella, or pavilion. It is even more important to wear protective clothing & apply sunscreen if there is no shade. Reflective surfaces like water, sand, snow, & concrete should also be avoided because they can reflect UV rays onto the skin, increasing exposure even in the presence of shade. UV rays can penetrate clouds & affect the skin even on overcast days, despite the widespread belief that they only harm the skin on sunny, warm days. For this reason, regardless of the weather, it is crucial to protect the skin from UV rays all year long. People who spend a lot of time in cars or close to windows at home or at work are still susceptible to UV damage because UV rays can also enter the body through windows. It is a misconception that darker skin tones are inherently shielded from the damaging effects of UV radiation, despite what some people think. Even though melanin in the skin offers some natural defence against UV radiation, people with darker skin are still susceptible to skin cancer, particularly in places where melanin levels are lower, like the palms of the hands, soles of the feet, & under the nails. Additionally, people with darker skin tones are less likely to exhibit obvious symptoms of sunburn, which may lead to them neglecting to take the necessary precautions against UV exposure. To lower the risk of skin damage & cancer, everyone should use sun protection techniques, regardless of skin type or colour. Avoiding tanning beds, which emit artificial UV radiation that can be even more concentrated than natural sunlight, is another important way to protect the skin from UV radiation. Particularly when used prior to the age of 35, tanning beds are linked to an elevated risk of melanoma, the most deadly type of skin cancer. Many people, particularly teenagers & young adults, use tanning beds to try to get a bronzed skin tone without realising that doing so greatly raises their risk of developing cancer. The World Health Organisation (WHO) has designated tanning beds as a Group 1 carcinogen, which means that they are known to cause cancer in humans, & their use has been associated with an increased risk of skin cancer. Many nations have enacted laws to limit access to tanning beds, especially for minors, as awareness of the risks associated with these devices has grown. Preventing skin cancer requires avoiding tanning beds & embracing a healthy, natural skin tone. Regular self-examinations of the skin are also essential for identifying any odd changes that might indicate the early stages of skin cancer. This entails keeping an eye out for asymmetry, uneven borders, colour variation, & changes in size or texture in moles & other areas. A healthcare professional should assess any questionable growths or changes; they may suggest additional testing or perform a biopsy. Successful treatment of skin cancer depends on early detection, & routinely examining the skin for anomalies can help spot possible problems before they worsen. People with certain risk factors, such as fair skin, a history of sunburns or excessive UV exposure, a compromised immune system, or a family history of skin cancer, should pay special attention to using sun protection to prevent skin cancer. Individuals who have these risk factors may need to take more drastic precautions against the sun & should be even more careful about shielding their skin from UV rays. Furthermore, it's critical to understand that lifetime exposure to UV light increases the risk of developing skin cancer. The risk increases with each incident of sunburn or unprotected sun exposure, & UV radiation damage may not always be obvious right away. Although the risk of skin cancer rises with age, UV exposure has long-lasting effects, so protecting the skin at a young age is essential to lowering the chance of getting skin cancer later in life. Reducing the incidence of skin cancer worldwide requires public health campaigns & educational initiatives that increase knowledge of the risks posed by UV rays, the value of sun protection, & the precautions people can take to protect their skin. In addition to teaching people about the dangers of UV exposure & the value of early detection, these campaigns can highlight the significance of using sunscreen, dressing in protective apparel, finding shade, & avoiding tanning beds. In addition to preventing skin cancer, shielding the skin from UV rays also helps avoid premature ageing, which is something that many people worry about. Wrinkles, sagging, & a decrease in skin elasticity are caused by UV radiation's acceleration of the skin's collagen & elastin fibre breakdown. Over time, people can maintain a healthier complexion & keep their skin looking young by using sun protection techniques. To sum up, shielding the skin from UV rays is essential for preserving general health & halting the growth of skin cancer & other skin-related disorders. The risk of skin damage & cancer can be considerably decreased by implementing a comprehensive approach to sun protection, which includes using sunscreen, wearing protective clothes, looking for shade, & staying away from tanning beds. In order to prevent skin cancer, it is essential to educate the public about the value of UV protection, encourage sun-safe practices, & support routine skin examinations. By working together, we can lessen the incidence of skin cancer & encourage better, more knowledgeable decisions about UV exposure.

Screening & Early Detection Strategies

In order to lower the mortality & morbidity linked to a variety of diseases, especially cancer, screening & early detection techniques are vital parts of contemporary healthcare. Early disease detection, frequently before symptoms show up, enables interventions that can greatly enhance prognosis, raise survival rates, & lessen the need for harsh treatments. One of the fundamental tenets of screening is that some illnesses, like cancer, frequently have a protracted latency period, during which time the patient or healthcare professional may not notice abnormal cells present. Therefore, the goal of early detection is to find these anomalies or risk factors as soon as possible. This can result in better outcomes, more efficient management, & earlier treatment. Screening is a key component of preventive healthcare since early detection of many cancers is linked to a marked decrease in death rates. Programs for cancer screening are usually created for groups that are more likely to get the disease because of things like age, genetic predisposition, lifestyle, & family history. Mammograms, for instance, are frequently used to detect breast cancer early, especially in women over 50 or those with a family history of the condition. Another important component of early detection is colorectal cancer screening; tests such as stool-based tests or colonoscopies are advised for people beginning at age 45, especially those with a family history or other risk factors. Similarly, depending on personal risk factors, women in their 20s or 30s should begin screening for cervical cancer, which is usually done by Pap smears or human papillomavirus (HPV) testing. Despite being debatable among some groups, lung cancer screening is becoming more & more advised for high-risk individuals, such as those who have smoked for a long time or have been exposed to environmental carcinogens. Screening aims to detect cancer or precancerous changes before they develop into more advanced, symptomatic stages, when there may be fewer & less effective treatment options. Accurately identifying individuals at risk, choosing suitable tests, & ensuring that people follow screening guidelines are all critical to the success of screening programs. Inaccurate results can result in missed diagnoses or needless procedures, so screening tools must be both sensitive & specific to reduce false positives & false negatives. The psychological effects of screening must also be taken into account because people may feel anxious or distressed about the possible outcomes. Even though screening programs frequently target cancer, early detection techniques can also be used for other illnesses, such as diabetes, heart disease, & infectious diseases like HIV & TB. Screening for cardiovascular disease entails keeping an eye on important risk factors like blood pressure, cholesterol, & glucose levels, which can reveal a person's propensity for heart disease & stroke. Interventions that can stop the development of more serious cardiovascular events, like heart attacks or strokes, are made possible by early detection of high blood pressure or elevated cholesterol levels. In a similar vein, diabetes screening is essential for detecting people with prediabetes or undiagnosed diabetes, which, if untreated, can result in major complications like kidney disease, neuropathy, & vision loss. Infectious disease screening can also stop the spread of disease & enable early treatment that can lessen complications & transmission, especially in high-risk groups. HIV screening, for instance, is now a standard component of preventive healthcare, particularly for those with risk factors like intravenous drug use or unprotected sex. Early HIV detection enables prompt antiretroviral therapy initiation, which can enhance quality of life & stop the development of AIDS. Beyond personal health, screening & early detection are crucial because they have important public health ramifications. By averting future, more costly, & intensive treatments, early detection & intervention can lower the overall burden of disease, enhance health outcomes, & save healthcare costs. Furthermore, in underprivileged or high-risk communities where access to healthcare may be restricted, early detection can aid in the identification of health disparities within populations. These populations can benefit from targeted screening programs that improve access to preventive care & address disparities in health outcomes. As genetic testing advances have the potential to identify people at higher risk for certain conditions even before symptoms or disease onset, the role of genomics & genetics in screening & early detection is rapidly changing. People who may have mutations in genes like BRCA1 & BRCA2, which are linked to an increased risk of breast &

ovarian cancers, can benefit from earlier intervention through genetic screening, especially for hereditary cancers. Preventive surgeries, more frequent screenings, or cancer-risk-lowering drugs may be part of early detection strategies for these people. Personalised medicine could greatly benefit from the incorporation of genetic testing into routine screening programs, which would allow medical professionals to customise prevention & treatment plans according to each patient's distinct genetic profile. Although genetic testing has a lot of promise, it also brings up ethical issues, such as privacy invasion, discrimination, & the psychological effects of being aware of one's genetic risks. The success of screening & early detection strategies depends heavily on public awareness & education in addition to technological advancements. People need to be made aware of the value of routine screening, the possible risks & advantages, & the suggested practices for different medical conditions. Public health campaigns, community organisations, & healthcare providers all have a significant impact on encouraging screening & teaching people how to identify risk factors & symptoms for conditions like diabetes, cancer, & heart disease. For people to be able to make educated decisions about their health & comprehend the importance of early detection, health literacy is essential. Early detection frequently makes the difference between life & death, especially in cases of cancer & other chronic illnesses that develop silently without showing any symptoms. Numerous studies demonstrate the advantages of early detection, demonstrating that cancers detected early have significantly higher survival rates than those detected at later stages. For example, early-stage breast cancer has a 5-year survival rate of over 90%, while metastatic breast cancer has a survival rate of less than 30%. Similar to this, colorectal cancer has a 5-year survival rate of over 90% if detected early; however, once the cancer has spread to other organs, survival rates sharply decline. These figures highlight how crucial early detection is to raising survival rates & lowering the burden of illness. The availability of tests & people's willingness to participate in these programs are both necessary for screening programs to be effective. Addressing obstacles like fear of the results, lack of access to healthcare, financial limitations, & linguistic or cultural differences is necessary to increase screening participation. Healthcare systems must implement measures that guarantee screening is available, reasonably priced, & culturally sensitive in order to get past these obstacles. Offering screenings at convenient locations, offering insurance coverage or financial aid, & utilising mobile health clinics to reach underprivileged populations are a few examples of how to do this. Emerging technologies like artificial intelligence (AI), machine learning, & digital health tools are starting to transform early detection strategies in addition to conventional screening techniques. In order to accurately identify early indicators of disease, AI & machine learning algorithms have demonstrated promise in the analysis of medical imaging, including mammograms, CT scans, & MRIs. These technologies have the potential to decrease human error, increase diagnostic accuracy, & produce faster results. Wearable technology & smartphone apps are examples of digital health tools that can track people's health in real time & provide early warning signs of possible problems. For example, wearable technology that monitors heart rate, activity, & sleep patterns can identify early indicators of diabetes or cardiovascular disease, encouraging people to consult a doctor before the condition worsens. The effectiveness of preventive healthcare can be further increased by incorporating AI & digital health technologies into screening & early detection programs. This will improve outcomes & lessen the burden of disease. There are still difficulties in putting screening & early detection techniques into practice globally, despite their advancements. Significant obstacles to screening exist in many low- & middle-income nations, such as inadequate access to diagnostic tools, a lack of qualified healthcare professionals, & a lack of a robust healthcare infrastructure. Innovative strategies like telemedicine, mobile health units, & community health workers can help close the gap & guarantee that screening reaches the people who need it most in these situations. Furthermore, international health agencies like the World Health Organisation (WHO) are crucial in promoting the growth of screening programs, especially for cancers that disproportionately impact people in areas with limited resources. It is impossible to overestimate the significance of screening & early detection in the battle against cancer & chronic illnesses. Screening saves lives & lessens the strain on healthcare systems by detecting diseases early, when they are most treatable. To ensure that everyone, regardless of age, background, or location, has access to the life-saving early detection services, screening programs must be improved & expanded through ongoing research, technological innovation, public education, & international collaboration.

Creating A Healthier Home Environment

Since the places we live in have a big influence on our physical, mental, & emotional health, making our homes healthier is crucial to fostering the wellbeing of both individuals & families. A home is a haven where people should feel safe, at ease, & encouraged to pursue healthy lifestyles. It is more than just a place to live. Reduced exposure to toxic substances, increased physical activity, a healthy diet, sound sleep, & mental well-being are all components of a healthy home environment. Through deliberate modifications to the home's physical, social, & emotional elements, people can establish a setting that enhances their general quality of life in addition to supporting their health. The removal or reduction of dangerous toxins & pollutants, which are frequently present in common household items, construction materials, & appliances, is one of the cornerstones of a healthier home. Common indoor pollutants like mould, radon, lead, pesticides, & volatile organic compounds (VOCs) can have a negative impact on health, especially for vulnerable groups like children, the elderly, & people with underlying medical conditions. Paints, cleaning supplies, air fresheners, &

some furniture materials, for example, release volatile organic compounds (VOCs). Prolonged exposure to these chemicals can cause headaches, respiratory problems, & even chronic illnesses like cancer. When remodelling or redecorating, homeowners can reduce these risks by using eco-friendly, non-toxic products like organic furniture made of non-toxic materials, low-VOC paints, & natural cleaning solutions. Making sure that homes are well-ventilated by installing air purifiers, using exhaust fans in bathrooms & kitchens, & opening windows frequently can greatly improve indoor air quality. Proper ventilation is also essential in minimising the accumulation of indoor air pollutants. Similarly, a healthy home environment depends on preventing mould growth through appropriate moisture control, which includes repairing leaks & installing dehumidifiers in damp areas like basements. Another important indoor pollutant associated with lung cancer is radon, an odourless & colourless gas that can seep into homes from the ground. Homeowners should test for radon levels, especially in areas where radon is known to be common. Children are particularly at risk for developmental delays & other severe health problems due to lead exposure, which can be caused by lead-based paint or plumbing systems in older homes. Maintaining a safe environment requires that homes constructed prior to 1978 be appropriately renovated & tested for lead hazards. Making design decisions that promote physical activity & decrease sedentary behaviours is another aspect of creating a healthier home, in addition to lowering environmental pollutants.

Family members can be encouraged to be more active by including areas for exercise, such as a yoga studio, home gym, or just a plain space for walking or stretching. Furthermore, establishing a welcoming outdoor area—whether by adding a patio, garden, or play area—can offer chances for outdoor leisure & exercise. In order to encourage more active lifestyles, indoor spaces should also be designed to encourage movement. For example, putting items in accessible areas to encourage walking, using standing desks instead of long periods of sitting, & adding stairs in multi-story homes. Actually, research indicates that when people live in a home that encourages movement, whether through visual cues or practical features, they are more likely to be physically active. Additionally, encouraging healthy eating practices is another aspect of a healthy home environment. In this sense, the kitchen is essential since it serves as the centre for preparing meals & storing food. Homeowners can prioritise kitchen organisation to make wholesome food easier to find & more convenient in order to promote healthier eating. This could entail minimising the amount of processed or unhealthy foods, keeping fresh fruits & vegetables in areas that are easily visible, & keeping healthy snacks close at hand. Additionally, meal preparation can be made simpler & more pleasurable by purchasing appliances like air fryers, food processors, & blenders that promote healthy cooking. Using cookware composed of non-toxic materials, like ceramic, cast iron, & stainless steel, can also lessen exposure to dangerous chemicals present in some nonstick coatings. Mindful eating, which entails paying attention to what one eats & taking the time to enjoy meals, is promoted by a healthier home environment. Making meals at home instead of ordering takeaway or fast food can also help people better manage their diet & stay away from unhealthy fats, sugar, & salt. Since sleep is essential for general health, making an environment that promotes sleep is equally important. Physical recuperation, mental clarity, emotional stability, & immune system health all depend on getting a good night's sleep. People can optimise their bedroom environment by creating a cool, dark, & quiet space to promote better sleep. This could entail utilising earplugs or white noise machines to minimise noise disruptions, blocking out light with blackout curtains, & adjusting the thermostat to a sleep-friendly setting, usually between 60 & 67 degrees Fahrenheit. For a good night's sleep, it's also critical to choose pillows that offer sufficient support & a comfortable mattress. Sleep hygiene techniques can also improve the quality of your sleep. These include keeping a regular sleep schedule, avoiding electronics right before bed, & doing peaceful things like reading or meditation. Other crucial tactics for guaranteeing restorative sleep include limiting exposure to blue light from screens prior to bed & steering clear of large meals or caffeine in the evening. A healthier home environment fosters mental & emotional well-being in addition to physical health. Family members should be able to unwind, rejuvenate, & partake in activities that promote relaxation & connection in the home, which should serve as an emotional haven. With neat, orderly areas that lessen chaos & clutter, the layout & design of the house have a big impact on fostering mental wellness. Because they can make one feel overwhelmed & impair concentration, cluttered spaces are frequently linked to higher stress levels. On the other hand, a neat, orderly environment fosters a sense of peace & order, making people feel less anxious & more in control. Since studies have shown that spending time in nature or just being surrounded by natural elements can lower stress & improve mood, incorporating elements of nature, such as houseplants, natural light, & outdoor views, can also contribute to emotional well-being. The benefits of the home for mental health are further increased by creating areas for social interaction, such as cosy seating areas for family get-togethers or spaces for hobbies & self-expression. The home should serve as a haven where people can relax & recharge in the fast-paced world of today, where maintaining a work-life balance can frequently be challenging. Additionally, cultivating wholesome relationships at home is just as crucial for mental well-being. Relationships can be strengthened & a loving, supportive environment can be created through open communication, shared activities, & family bonding, all of which support mental wellness. Setting limits & respecting personal time & space are also crucial for preserving peaceful relationships & avoiding interpersonal stress in homes where families or roommates share space. Reducing digital distractions & encouraging thoughtful technology use are further aspects of creating a healthier home environment. With the widespread use of smartphones, tablets, & other gadgets, excessive screen time can disrupt social interactions, sleep patterns, & physical activity, which can have detrimental effects on one's physical & mental well-being. Reducing screen time, particularly before bed or during meals, can improve sleep patterns & foster deeper relationships with family members. A clearer separation between work & home life can also be achieved by allocating specific areas for study or work, away from areas for leisure. This will lower stress levels & increase productivity. Lastly, cultivating a sense of community & environmental responsibility is a component of making the home healthier. Making deliberate choices to cut back on waste, save energy, & lessen one's carbon footprint not only helps the environment but also provides a sustainable living model for the family. In addition to lowering utility costs, recycling, composting, & the use of energy-efficient appliances can lessen the household's environmental effect. Reducing exposure to hazardous chemicals & encouraging a more ecologically conscious lifestyle can also be achieved by selecting eco-friendly materials like wood that has been sourced sustainably, recycled textiles, & non-toxic cleaning supplies. In conclusion, making deliberate decisions that put physical, mental, & emotional well-being first is necessary to create a healthier home environment. People can create an environment that supports their general well-being by lowering their exposure to toxins, encouraging physical activity, developing healthy eating habits, facilitating restful sleep, & cultivating positive relationships. Additionally, a healthy home environment can support feelings of security, comfort, & belonging—all of which are essential for living a happy & balanced life. People can make their homes healthier, more nurturing spaces that promote a life of vitality & wellness by making small adjustments & thoughtful choices.

CHAPTER 5: EVIDENCE-BASED APPROACHES TO PREVENTION

Because they provide scientifically proven strategies that can dramatically lower the risk of disease onset & enhance health outcomes for all populations, evidence-based approaches to prevention are essential in the fight against diseases like cancer, cardiovascular disease, & chronic conditions. In order to ensure that health interventions are both successful & long-lasting in preventing disease, these methods rely on an abundance of thorough research & clinical data. Health professionals can find preventive measures that not only work but also have long-term advantages by looking at large-scale studies, randomised controlled trials, & meta-analyses. This will lessen the need for future invasive & expensive treatments. The scientific method, which includes developing hypotheses, carrying out experiments, & evaluating the outcomes to make judgements regarding the effectiveness of particular health interventions, is the cornerstone of evidence-based prevention. Evidence-based prevention places a lot of emphasis on lifestyle modification, which includes adjustments to stress management, physical activity, food, & alcohol & cigarette use. It is commonly acknowledged that these factors are the primary causes of chronic illnesses like obesity, diabetes, heart disease, & cancer. Numerous chronic conditions can be avoided or their onset can be lessened by adopting healthy habits, such as eating a balanced diet full of fruits, vegetables, whole grains, & lean proteins & getting regular exercise. For instance, research indicates that people who combine strength training activities with at least 150 minutes of moderate-intensity aerobic exercise each week are less likely to suffer from heart disease, stroke, & some cancers, such as lung, breast, & colorectal cancer. Additionally, one of the best strategies to avoid obesity-related conditions like type 2 diabetes & hypertension—which are significant risk factors for cardiovascular disease & some types of cancer—is to maintain a healthy weight through a balanced diet & regular exercise. By emphasising whole, plant-based foods, healthy fats, & lean proteins, evidence-based dietary approaches—like the Mediterranean diet—have been demonstrated to enhance cardiovascular health & lower the risk of cancer. However, eating too much red meat, processed foods, & sugary drinks is linked to a higher risk of developing a number of chronic illnesses. Another essential component of evidence-based prevention, in addition to healthy eating & exercise, is quitting smoking. Worldwide, smoking is the primary preventable cause of respiratory illnesses, cardiovascular disease, & cancer. Studies have shown that even modest smoking cessation can have a major positive impact on one's health. Numerous studies have demonstrated the effectiveness of programs & interventions that promote quitting smoking, including behavioural counselling, nicotine replacement therapy, & medication. The risk of heart disease, stroke, lung cancer, & other chronic conditions can actually be significantly decreased by quitting smoking at any age, according to research. Additionally, excessive alcohol use is a known risk factor for a number of cancers, such as esophageal, breast, & liver cancer. Public health recommendations to limit alcohol intake are based on the evidence that even moderate alcohol consumption can raise the risk of cancer. The best way to reduce the risk of cancer for people who don't drink alcohol is to abstain completely, according to the evidence. Evidence-based tactics that highlight the long-term advantages of prevention & the significance of early intervention are the foundation of public health campaigns, such as those that target smoking & excessive drinking. Implementing screening & early detection programs is another essential component of evidence-based prevention. It has been demonstrated that by enabling prompt & less invasive treatments, these programs—which concentrate on identifying diseases at an early, asymptomatic stage—reduce mortality rates. By detecting precancerous changes or early-stage cancers that can be effectively treated, routine screenings for breast cancer using mammography, colorectal cancer using colonoscopy, & cervical cancer using Pap smears or HPV testing, for instance, have been demonstrated to lower mortality rates. Additionally, there is evidence to support the use of genetic screening to find people who might be more susceptible to certain cancers or inherited conditions. This enables targeted interventions & early preventive measures. However, the benefits & risks of early detection must be carefully considered, & screening recommendations must be supported by strong evidence. Although screening can save lives, there are risks associated with it, including overdiagnosis, needless procedures, & false positives, all of which need to be considered when developing screening programs. Another area where evidence-based practices have been extremely helpful in preventing infectious diseases & some forms of cancer is vaccination. Extensive clinical trials & research have supported the development of vaccines for diseases like influenza, liver cancer (hepatitis B vaccine), & cervical cancer (HPV vaccine), demonstrating a significant decrease in the incidence of these diseases among vaccinated populations. For instance, the HPV vaccine is now commonly advised for adolescents as part of regular vaccination schedules due to its demonstrated high effectiveness in preventing cervical & other cancers linked to HPV infection. It has been demonstrated that the flu vaccine lowers the risk of influenza-related complications, hospitalisations, & fatalities, especially in susceptible groups like the elderly & people with long-term medical conditions. One of the most economical public health measures for preventing disease & lessening the strain on healthcare systems is vaccination campaigns, especially in high-risk communities. Evidence-based approaches to prevention include environmental strategies that aim to reduce exposure to environmental pollutants & carcinogens, in addition to behavioural, lifestyle, & vaccination interventions. Public health initiatives to reduce exposure to chemicals like radiation, pesticides, asbestos, & air pollution have been prompted by scientific evidence linking environmental factors to cancer risk. Long-term exposure to air pollution, especially fine particulate matter, has been linked to an increased risk of lung cancer & other cancers as well as respiratory illnesses. Evidence-based prevention strategies must include measures to improve air quality, such as promoting clean energy sources, regulating emissions, & planning cities. In a similar vein, measures to curtail the use of pesticides, especially in agricultural operations, have been connected to decreased incidence of some types of cancer, such as those brought on by exposure to the common herbicide glyphosate. With laws limiting exposure to dangerous chemicals, carcinogens, & physical agents at work dramatically lowering the risk of occupational cancers, occupational health & safety plays a critical role in evidence-based prevention as well. Stricter workplace safety regulations have been shown to reduce cancer rates among exposed workers, according to research supporting their implementation. This highlights the significance of public health interventions grounded in solid scientific evidence. Furthermore, promoting long-term health & well-being requires establishing healthier settings in communities, workplaces, & schools through laws that support mental wellness, physical activity, & a balanced diet. Evidence-based prevention also applies to mental health, where strategies that lessen stress, increase resilience, & strengthen social ties are essential for averting mental health illnesses & stress-related chronic conditions. The increasing amount of research on social support networks, mindfulness, & cognitive-behavioral therapy has shown how successful these interventions are at preventing mental health problems & lessening the negative physiological effects of long-term stress. For instance, it has been demonstrated that mindfulness-based stress reduction (MBSR) lowers stress, anxiety, & depression while also enhancing general quality of life & possibly lowering the risk of stress-related illnesses like autoimmune diseases & cardiovascular disease. Furthermore, since people with strong social ties typically experience lower stress levels & better mental health outcomes, social support is essential to mental wellness. In order to promote a sense of belonging & emotional well-being, evidence-based interventions that encourage social engagement, community building, & access to mental health resources are crucial. To sum up, evidence-based prevention strategies are critical to lowering the prevalence of chronic illnesses, enhancing public health, & building healthier communities. These tactics, which are based on thorough scientific research & clinical data, offer tried-&-true ways to promote healthy lifestyles, prevent illness, & lessen the toll that disease takes on both people & healthcare systems. Evidence-based prevention strategies provide a thorough & multidimensional approach to protecting health, ranging from lifestyle interventions like diet & exercise to screening programs, vaccinations, environmental policies, & mental health support. Reducing the worldwide burden of disease, enhancing health equity, & guaranteeing a healthier future for everybody will depend on sustained investment in research, public health initiatives, & evidence-based policy implementation.

The Latest Research In Cancer Prevention

Recent advances in cancer prevention research have produced ground-breaking findings & improved methods for reducing the risk of getting the disease, giving people & communities a new lease on life. Scientists now have a better understanding of the intricate interactions between genetics, environment, & lifestyle factors that lead to the development of cancer thanks to developments in molecular biology, genomics, & epidemiology. Precision medicine, which attempts to customise preventative measures according to a person's genetic composition, environmental exposures, & lifestyle decisions, is gaining more & more attention from researchers. The emergence of cancer risk prediction models that combine behavioural, environmental, & genetic factors to more accurately identify people at high risk for particular cancer types is one of the most exciting advancements in cancer prevention. More individualised approaches to prevention are made possible by these models, such as focused lifestyle modifications & early screening techniques that can identify precancerous alterations before they progress to cancer. With the discovery of more genetic markers & mutations that predispose people to specific cancers, including breast, ovarian, colorectal, & prostate cancer, research on the role of genetics in cancer prevention has advanced significantly. As a result, genetic screening programs have been established, allowing people with a genetic or family history of cancer to get regular screenings & take preventative actions like chemoprevention or prophylactic surgery. For example, oophorectomies, mastectomies, & chemopreventive drugs like tamoxifen, which have been demonstrated to reduce cancer risk in high-risk groups, are now available to women who have BRCA1 or BRCA2 gene mutations, which greatly raise the risk of breast & ovarian cancer. The role of lifestyle factors, including diet, physical activity, alcohol consumption, smoking, & sleep, in modifying cancer risk is another area of intense focus in cancer prevention. A balanced diet full of fruits, vegetables, whole grains, & lean proteins, along with regular exercise & maintaining a healthy weight, have been repeatedly demonstrated to significantly lower the risk of developing colorectal, breast, & lung cancers, among other cancers. Increased physical activity, for instance, has been linked to a 20% lower risk of breast cancer & a lower risk of other cancers, including colon & endometrial cancer. Furthermore, a lower risk of cancer & improved general health outcomes have been linked to dietary patterns like the Mediterranean diet, which places an emphasis on plant-based foods, healthy fats, & lean proteins. Numerous studies have also been conducted on the function of particular dietary components, including fibre, antioxidants, & phytonutrients. Consuming a wide range of vibrant fruits & vegetables, which are high in vitamins, minerals, & phytochemicals, has been shown to improve the body's natural defences against cancer by scavenging free radicals & lowering oxidative stress, which is a process connected to the development of cancer cells. Compounds in cruciferous vegetables, like Brussels sprouts, kale, & broccoli, in particular, have demonstrated promise in stopping the growth of cancer cells & causing precancerous cells to undergo apoptosis, or programmed cell death. On the other hand, since processed foods, red meat, & sugary drinks are associated with obesity, chronic inflammation, & alterations in metabolic function that can lead to the development of cancer, limiting them has been shown to reduce the risk of developing cancer. One of the biggest modifiable risk factors for cancer is still smoking, & the most recent research keeps highlighting how crucial quitting smoking is to preventing cancer. According to studies, smoking cessation at any age can dramatically lower the risk of lung cancer as well as other smoking-related cancers like head & neck, bladder, & esophageal cancers. According to studies on the mechanisms underlying tobacco-induced carcinogenesis, smoking causes immune suppression, DNA mutations, & chronic inflammation, all of which foster the growth of cancer. However, quitting smoking can have major health benefits, including a significant reduction in the risk of cancer over time, even for those who have smoked for many years. The worldwide burden of tobacco-related cancers has decreased in large part due to efforts to lower smoking rates through public health campaigns, smoking cessation programs, & tobacco product regulation. Another known risk factor for a number of cancers, such as colorectal, breast, & liver cancer, is alcohol use. Recent studies have further demonstrated that alcohol is a carcinogen & that moderate alcohol use raises the risk of developing cancer. Research has demonstrated that alcohol-induced carcinogenesis happens via a number of pathways, such as the breakdown of folate metabolism, which is crucial for cell division & DNA repair, & the conversion of ethanol to acetaldehyde, a poisonous substance that can harm DNA. Public health groups now advise reducing alcohol intake to lower the risk of cancer, with some recommendations stating that people should abstain from alcohol completely for the best chance of preventing cancer. The role of immunological dysfunction & chronic inflammation in the development of cancer has also been the subject of recent studies. One of the main causes of cancer progression has been found to be chronic inflammation, which is frequently connected to lifestyle choices like smoking, obesity, & poor diet. In addition to preventing apoptosis & fostering the survival & growth of cancer cells, inflammation can also produce an environment that facilitates tumour growth & metastasis. As possible cancer prevention measures, researchers are looking into anti-inflammatory treatments like non-steroidal anti-inflammatory drugs (NSAIDs) & specific dietary supplements. However, because these interventions can have adverse effects, their long-term use needs to be carefully balanced. Vaccine use is another exciting area of cancer prevention research. It has been demonstrated that vaccination against viruses that cause cancer, such as the hepatitis B virus (HBV) & the human papillomavirus (HPV), greatly lowers the risk of liver, cervical, & other cancers linked to these infections. For instance, it has been shown that the HPV vaccine can prevent most cervical cancers & other cancers linked to HPV, including vulvar, oropharyngeal, & anal cancers. Similarly, the HBV vaccine is very successful in preventing chronic hepatitis B infection-related liver cancer. The global incidence of cancer could be decreased by the widespread use of these vaccines, especially in nations where viral infections are prevalent. Other vaccines that target tumor-associated antigens & the creation of therapeutic cancer vaccines that might aid the immune system in identifying & eliminating cancer cells are also being studied for their potential role in cancer prevention. Microbiome science, which investigates how the gut microbiota affects cancer risk, is another fascinating area of cancer prevention research. According to recent research, dysbiosis, or an imbalance in the gut microbiome, can cause immunological dysfunction, inflammation, & changes in metabolic processes that may encourage the growth of cancer. These days, research is concentrating on how the gut microbiota affects the development of cancers like colorectal cancer & whether probiotics, prebiotics, & dietary modifications can help restore a healthy microbiome & lower the risk of developing cancer. Additionally, the gut microbiota is a promising area for personalised cancer prevention & treatment because of growing evidence that it interacts with the immune system & the body's reaction to cancer therapies. Preventing cancer has also shown promise thanks to precision medicine, which customises prevention & treatment plans based on a person's genetic, environmental, & lifestyle data. Researchers are enhancing our capacity to prevent cancer in high-risk populations by identifying genetic mutations that raise the risk of the disease & customising preventive measures, such as more frequent screenings, lifestyle changes, or prophylactic treatments. Targeted therapies that can stop cancer from starting or spreading in people with particular genetic profiles have already been developed as a result of advancements in genetic testing & personalised medicine. The effect of environmental factors, such as pesticides, air pollution, & occupational hazards, on cancer risk is a significant area of research in cancer prevention. According to studies, people who live or work in areas with high pollution levels or who are exposed to certain carcinogens at work may be more likely to develop cancer as a result of environmental exposure to carcinogenic chemicals. With public health policies aimed at lowering air pollution, controlling chemical exposure, & supporting cleaner energy sources, research into lowering environmental exposures & establishing safer work environments is essential to cancer prevention. Lastly, one of the most important aspects of cancer prevention is still early detection. Early cancer detection could be greatly aided by developments in screening technologies, such as liquid biopsies, which identify genetic material linked to cancer in the blood. Even before symptoms show up, liquid biopsies may make it possible to identify cancers in their earliest, most curable stages. The accuracy &

effectiveness of cancer screenings could be increased by other developments, such as AI-driven imaging technologies, which would make it simpler to spot tumours or precancerous changes early on. In summary, recent studies on cancer prevention have advanced significantly in a number of areas, including genetics, lifestyle changes, vaccinations, & early detection tools. These developments present fresh chances to lower the prevalence of cancer, enhance preventative measures, & eventually save lives. Even though there has been a lot of progress, more study & funding are needed to improve our knowledge of cancer prevention & create more individualised & efficient plans that can be used with people of all risk levels. The increasing amount of data offers a solid basis for a future in which cancer prevention is not only feasible but also available to everyone, lowering the global cancer burden & enhancing public health results.

Integrative Medicine: What Works & What Doesn't

Integrative medicine seeks to treat the full person, addressing physical, emotional, & spiritual well-being in order to promote optimal health. It does this by combining traditional medical treatments with complementary therapies. Because more people are interested in learning how these complementary therapies can be successfully incorporated into conventional medical procedures, this holistic approach has become increasingly popular. It is based on the notion that a mix of traditional & alternative therapies can speed up the healing process & raise general quality of life, particularly when it comes to managing pain, chronic illnesses, & side effects from cancer treatment. Though there is no denying integrative medicine's appeal, there is still continuous discussion regarding what works, what doesn't, & the best way to incorporate evidence-based practices into healthcare. The focus on patient-centered care—that is, treatment plans that are customised to the needs, preferences, & values of the individual—is a fundamental tenet of integrative medicine. This frequently includes treatments that are thought to improve the body's capacity for healing & alleviate symptoms, such as acupuncture, massage, herbal medicine, yoga, meditation, & nutritional supplements. To lessen symptoms, speed up recovery, & encourage the body's inherent healing processes, these therapies are frequently combined with more conventional treatments like surgery, chemotherapy, or medicine. The goal is to enhance patient outcomes by using them in conjunction with scientifically proven therapies, not in place of traditional medical treatments. Acupuncture, for instance, is frequently used to treat pain & alleviate side effects from chemotherapy, such as fatigue & nausea. Although results can vary greatly & further research is required to pinpoint the precise mechanisms underlying its efficacy, studies have indicated that acupuncture may offer a modest benefit in lowering pain & enhancing the general quality of life for cancer patients. Similarly, it has been demonstrated that yoga & mindfulness meditation can help cancer patients & people with chronic pain manage stress, lower anxiety, & encourage relaxation, thereby enhancing their mental & emotional health. However, not all complementary therapies have shown the same level of efficacy, & there is conflicting scientific evidence for some of these practices. For instance, plants & plant-based compounds are frequently praised for their health benefits in herbal medicine, a popular therapy in integrative medicine. Nevertheless, little is known about the effectiveness & safety of many herbal remedies. Certain herbs, like turmeric & ginger, have been demonstrated to possess antioxidant & anti-inflammatory qualities, making them useful for treating symptoms like inflammation or nausea. However, some herbs, like St. John's Wort, can interact with prescription drugs & cause harm, particularly if not properly monitored. The use of herbal remedies in integrative medicine is severely hampered by the lack of standardisation in their preparation & dosage as well as the inconsistent quality of the products. Additionally, despite the fact that many patients report benefits from herbal supplements, the safety profiles of these treatments are still being investigated, & there may not be enough data to support their widespread clinical use. Nutritional therapy, which incorporates diet & supplements into treatment plans to improve health outcomes, is another area of integrative medicine. Research continuously demonstrates that a balanced diet full of fruits, vegetables, whole grains, & lean proteins can lower the risk of cancer, heart disease, &

other chronic conditions. Nutrition is unquestionably important for maintaining general health & preventing disease. Probiotics, vitamin D, & omega-3 fatty acids are a few supplements that have drawn interest due to their possible health advantages. For instance, omega-3 fatty acids have anti-inflammatory qualities & may help lower the risk of heart disease & some types of cancer. However, because there is little to no evidence to support the use of many other supplements, like multivitamins, in preventing chronic diseases, their benefits are still debatable. Furthermore, excessive consumption of some vitamins & minerals may be hazardous, resulting in toxicity or adverse drug interactions. Therefore, even though certain supplements & dietary changes may be beneficial for certain people, their use needs to be cautious & supervised by a healthcare provider to guarantee their efficacy & safety. Another topic of intense interest is the function of mind-body therapies in integrative medicine. Deep breathing techniques, yoga, & meditation are common methods for reducing stress, improving relaxation, & fostering serenity. These methods are useful for managing chronic illnesses & preventing disease because they have been demonstrated to enhance emotional well-being, lessen anxiety, & lower blood pressure. Specifically, the ability of mindfulness-based stress reduction (MBSR) to lessen the symptoms of chronic pain, depression, & anxiety has drawn a lot of attention. Research indicates that MBSR can enhance general quality of life while assisting patients in managing the psychological toll of illnesses like cancer, heart disease, & chronic pain. Even though a lot of patients report good results, the scientific evidence for these treatments is not always strong, & individual results can vary & occasionally show only slight effects. Making sure complementary therapies don't conflict with traditional medical treatments is a major challenge in integrative medicine. Prescription drugs & some alternative therapies, especially those that use supplements, may interact negatively, decreasing the effectiveness of the former or producing negative side effects. For instance, some supplements & herbs may conflict with blood thinners, chemotherapy, or high blood pressure drugs. Therefore, to guarantee that all treatments function safely & synergistically, integrative medicine necessitates tight coordination between medical professionals. Carefully weighing the advantages & disadvantages of complementary therapies is frequently necessary when integrating them into traditional medical care. To make sure complementary therapies are safe & don't interfere with other treatments, patients should always talk to their healthcare providers about any complementary therapies they want to try. Patients & providers must be well-informed because it can be difficult to distinguish between therapies that have been shown to be effective & those that are more anecdotal in nature. Sometimes, especially when dealing with conditions like cancer or chronic pain, patients may be looking for alternative therapies because they are unhappy with traditional treatments. Integrative medicine gives patients more choices & a sense of empowerment, but it's important to make sure they don't choose risky, unproven treatments over evidence-based ones. In order to balance the need for scientific rigour with the desire for holistic care, education is crucial in assisting patients in making well-informed decisions about their treatment options. All things considered, when applied properly, integrative medicine has a great deal of promise to enhance health outcomes. Particularly in the areas of symptom management, mental health improvement, & general well-being enhancement, complementary therapies such as acupuncture, massage therapy, yoga, meditation, & nutritional support can offer significant advantages. Differentiating between treatments that have solid scientific support & those that haven't shown consistent or proven efficacy is still difficult, though. Healthcare professionals must give evidence-based practices top priority as integrative medicine develops in order to guarantee that patients receive the best care possible while lowering needless risks. To guide the integration of complementary therapies into clinical settings, thorough research & clinical trials are required to assess their safety & efficacy. Integrative medicine has the potential to provide a genuinely individualised, patient-centered approach to care that improves quality of life & health outcomes as more solid evidence becomes available. In the end, integrative medicine should be used with an open mind but carefully weighed against professional advice & scientific data to make sure it complements traditional medical treatments rather than takes their place.

The Role Of Supplements In Cancer Risk Reduction

As more people look for ways to reduce their risk of cancer through nutritional interventions, the role of supplements in cancer risk reduction has become a hotly debated topic in the scientific & medical communities. Vitamins, minerals, & other natural substances found in supplements are frequently thought of as an easy & quick way to prevent cancer & enhance health. Because the effectiveness of supplements in lowering cancer risk depends on a number of factors, such as the type of supplement, dosage, individual genetic predispositions, & the presence of other lifestyle factors like diet, exercise, & environmental exposures, research in this area is intricate & multifaceted. The idea that certain vitamins & minerals are essential for immune system support, oxidative damage prevention, & normal cellular function—all of which are critical for cancer prevention—gives supplements the potential to lower cancer risk. Although some supplements have demonstrated promise in lowering the risk of cancer, there is still conflicting evidence to support their widespread use, & many supplements' safety & effectiveness are questioned, particularly when taken in large quantities or in conjunction with other medical interventions. Antioxidants, which include vitamins A, C, & E, as well as selenium & other trace minerals, are one of the supplement categories that have been studied the most in relation to cancer prevention. Free radicals are unstable molecules that can harm DNA & cause mutations, which are a defining feature of cancer. Antioxidants are believed to neutralise these molecules. The body naturally sustains damage from free radicals as a result of metabolic processes & environmental factors like smoking, pollution, & UV radiation. Antioxidants have been promoted as a possible way to lower the risk of cancer because oxidative stress is thought to play a role in the development of several cancer types. For example, vitamin C, a strong antioxidant, has been researched for its capacity to lower inflammation & shield cells from oxidative damage, two processes that contribute to the development of cancer. Vitamin C may reduce the risk of some cancers, including esophageal & stomach cancer, according to some preliminary research. Subsequent clinical trials, however, have produced conflicting findings; some indicate that vitamin C has no benefit in lowering the incidence of cancer, while others point to a possible role for the vitamin in lessening the severity of cancer symptoms or enhancing treatment outcomes, especially when combined with traditional therapies. Comparably, a number of studies have examined vitamin E, another antioxidant, for its potential to lower the risk of prostate & lung cancer, with varying degrees of success. Concerns have been raised that high doses of vitamin E may actually increase the risk of certain cancers or interfere with the effectiveness of chemotherapy, despite some studies suggesting that vitamin E supplementation may lower cancer risk, especially in people with low dietary intake of this vitamin. This emphasises how crucial it is to take supplements sparingly & under a doctor's supervision. A trace mineral with antioxidant qualities, selenium has also been researched for its possible role in preventing cancer, specifically colorectal, lung, & prostate cancers. Interest in selenium as a cancer prevention agent has grown as a result of some extensive studies, including the Nutritional Prevention of Cancer (NPC) trial, which found that selenium supplementation was linked to a lower incidence of prostate cancer. The long-term safety & effectiveness of selenium supplementation, however, have been called into question by other research, & some have expressed worries that high doses of selenium may be toxic. These results highlight the need for additional study to establish the ideal dosage & length of time for selenium supplementation in the prevention of cancer. In addition to antioxidants, other supplements have been investigated for possible cancer-preventive qualities. For instance, vitamin D, which is essential for calcium balance & bone health, has drawn interest due to its potential to lower the risk of several cancers, such as prostate, colon, & breast cancer. Sunlight exposure causes the skin to produce vitamin D, & many people have low vitamin D levels as a result of insufficient sun exposure, particularly in colder climates or among people who spend a lot of time indoors. Some research indicates that vitamin D supplementation may lower cancer risk by promoting normal cell growth, regulating immune function, & inhibiting cancer cell proliferation. Studies have shown that low levels of vitamin D are linked to an increased risk of certain cancers. For example, observational studies suggest a protective effect against breast cancer, & clinical trials have suggested that vitamin D supplementation may lower the risk of colorectal cancer. The evidence is still conflicting, though, with some studies finding no discernible benefit & high vitamin D dosages possibly having negative side effects like kidney damage or hypercalcemia. It has also been investigated how omega-3 fatty acids, which are present in fish oil & some plant-based sources, may help prevent cancer. Chronic inflammation is a known risk factor for cancer, & omega-3 fatty acids are well known for their anti-inflammatory qualities. In lab experiments, omega-3 fatty acids have been demonstrated to lower inflammation, alter immune responses, & stop the growth of cancer cells. According to certain observational studies, consuming more omega-3 fatty acids may lower the risk of developing cancers like colorectal, prostate, & breast cancer. Clinical trial findings, however, have been conflicting; some research indicates that omega-3 supplementation does not significantly lower the risk of cancer, while other studies point to possible advantages. Variations in study design, participant characteristics, & omega-3 dosages may be the cause of these discrepancies. Green tea extract, garlic, folic acid, & curcumin—the active ingredient in turmeric—are other supplements that have been studied for their potential to prevent cancer. A B vitamin called folic acid is essential for DNA synthesis & repair. According to some research, consuming enough folate may lower the risk of colorectal cancer by preventing DNA damage. The evidence is conflicting, though, & some research has expressed worries that taking too many supplements containing folate may encourage the growth of cancer cells that already exist. The potential of green tea extract, which contains catechins with anti-inflammatory & antioxidant qualities, to lower the risk of breast, prostate, & colorectal cancer has been investigated. Clinical trials have produced conflicting findings, with some indicating no discernible influence on cancer risk, despite laboratory research suggesting that green tea extract may suppress the growth of cancer cells & trigger apoptosis (programmed cell death). Known for its antioxidant & anti-inflammatory properties, curcumin has demonstrated promise in lab studies as a possible cancer preventive agent, especially for digestive tract cancers like stomach & colon cancer. Curcumin's bioavailability is restricted, though, & further study is required to ascertain its efficacy in people. Garlic has long been linked to a number of health advantages, including a lower risk of cancer. By strengthening the immune system & preventing the growth of cancer cells, garlic consumption may lower the risk of some cancers, including colorectal, esophageal, & stomach cancer, according to some research. More research is necessary to elucidate the possible role of garlic supplements in cancer prevention, as the evidence is still inconclusive. Although some supplements may help lower the risk of cancer, it's crucial to understand that no single supplement can ensure cancer prevention & that they shouldn't be used in place of a balanced diet, frequent exercise, & other preventive measures. Moreover, there are risks associated with high supplement dosages, particularly when taken for prolonged periods of time. These risks include toxicity, nutrient imbalances, & interactions with other medications or treatments. Therefore, the role of supplements in preventing cancer should be viewed in the context of a balanced lifestyle. Before beginning any supplementation program, people should speak with their healthcare providers, especially if they are receiving treatment for cancer or have underlying medical conditions. Much of the research on supplements & cancer prevention is still in progress, & the available data is far from definitive. The best way to lower the risk of cancer is still to combine good eating practices, frequent exercise, quitting smoking, & wearing enough sunscreen, even though some supplements may have slight advantages. To define the best dosages, ascertain the long-term safety of supplementation, & elucidate the mechanisms by which supplements may affect cancer risk, more research is required. In the interim, people must use supplements with caution & rely on tried-&-true, evidence-based cancer prevention techniques while also keeping up with new developments in the field.

Addressing Genetic Risks Through Lifestyle Choices

As researchers continue to examine how a person's genetic composition interacts with environmental &

behavioural factors to influence the development of diseases, including cancer, addressing genetic risks through lifestyle choices is a new area of study in cancer prevention. Although a person's susceptibility to some types of cancer is certainly influenced by their genetic makeup, lifestyle decisions such as food, exercise, & exposure to environmental pollutants can significantly reduce these risks. The significance of comprehending genetic susceptibilities to cancer has been emphasised by developments in genomics & personalised medicine; however, they also emphasise that fate is not solely determined by genetics. Rather, lifestyle factors are becoming more widely acknowledged for their capacity to alter the influence of genetic risks, providing a way for those with a higher genetic risk to actively lower their risk of cancer. One of the most important discoveries in the field of cancer prevention is that, regardless of a person's genetic predisposition, lifestyle choices may be able to prevent up to 70% of cancer cases. This offers a positive outlook since it implies that proactive lifestyle modifications can lower risk even for people with a family history of cancer or certain genetic mutations, such as those linked to colorectal cancer (e.g., Lynch syndrome) or breast cancer (e.g., BRCA1 & BRCA2). Regardless of a person's genetic background, diet, exercise, & maintaining a healthy weight are some of the most significant factors that can affect their risk of developing cancer. Maintaining optimal cellular function & bolstering the body's natural defence mechanisms require a diet rich in nutrients & well-balanced. Studies have indicated that diets high in fruits, vegetables, whole grains, lean meats, & healthy fats can lower the risk of a number of cancers, such as breast, prostate, & colorectal cancer. For instance, because of its anti-inflammatory qualities & capacity to promote healthy metabolic processes, the Mediterranean diet—which is rich in fruits, vegetables, olive oil, & seafood—has been linked to a lower risk of cancer & other chronic illnesses. On the other hand, a higher risk of cancer, especially colorectal cancer, has been associated with diets heavy in processed foods, red meat, & sugary drinks. There is also ongoing research on the role of particular nutrients, including fibre, antioxidants, vitamins, & minerals, in preventing cancer. Because it promotes a healthy gut microbiome, inhibits the production of carcinogenic compounds, & helps maintain a healthy digestive system, fiber—found in plant-based foods like fruits, vegetables, & whole grains—is especially crucial in lowering the risk of colorectal cancer. Vitamins C & E are examples of antioxidants that are thought to shield cells from oxidative damage, which can result in DNA mutations & the development of cancer. By promoting immunological function, controlling cell division, & lowering inflammation, other nutrients, such as vitamin D & omega-3 fatty acids, have also been linked to a lower risk of cancer. Since regular physical activity has been demonstrated to lower the risk of several cancer types, including breast, colon, & endometrial cancer, exercise & physical activity are also important factors in lowering cancer risk. Exercise aids in controlling hormone levels, including insulin & oestrogen, which, when present in excess, are linked to an increased risk of developing some types of cancer. In addition, exercise lowers inflammation, boosts the immune system, & encourages healthy weight management—all of which are critical for preventing cancer. A lower risk of cancer has been linked to even moderate physical activity, like walking or cycling, underscoring the significance of integrating movement into daily life. Regular exercise can have a protective effect for people with a higher genetic risk for cancer, reducing some of the elevated risks brought on by their genetic predisposition. Another important factor that affects cancer risk is obesity, as there is mounting evidence that excess body fat increases the risk of developing several cancers, such as pancreatic, liver, & breast cancer. Hormones & inflammatory chemicals produced by adipose tissue, especially visceral fat, have the potential to stimulate the growth of cancer cells. For this reason, maintaining a healthy weight through diet & exercise is crucial to preventing cancer, especially in those with genetic risk factors. By lowering insulin resistance, controlling hormone levels, & enhancing general metabolic health, maintaining a healthy weight can help lower the risk of cancer. Reducing the risk of cancer requires addressing two modifiable lifestyle factors that are directly associated with an increased risk: smoking & alcohol consumption. About 30% of all cancer-related deaths, especially those from lung cancer, are caused by smoking, which is the primary preventable cause of cancer. Smoking damages DNA, increases inflammation, & impairs immunity, all of which are factors in the development of cancer. The negative effects of smoking are especially dangerous for people who have a genetic predisposition to lung cancer, such as those who have specific genetic mutations or a family history of the disease. One of the best strategies to lower your risk of developing cancer is to stop smoking, & even long-time smokers can benefit from quitting. Drinking alcohol increases the risk of developing liver, breast, & colorectal cancers, among other cancers. Long-term alcohol consumption can raise the body's insulin & oestrogen levels, which are both associated with the development of cancer. Reducing alcohol consumption or abstaining completely is a crucial cancer risk reduction strategy for people with genetic mutations or a family history of alcohol-related cancers. Environmental exposures are important in preventing cancer in addition to these main lifestyle factors. A key component of lowering the risk of cancer is avoiding dangerous toxins & carcinogens, such as those present in pollution, tobacco smoke, & specific chemicals in household goods. Reducing exposure to environmental carcinogens can further lower the risk of cancer in people with genetic predispositions. For instance, people with a genetic predisposition to skin cancer should be careful about sun protection & stay away from excessive UV radiation, while those with a family history of lung cancer should avoid secondhand smoke exposure. The study of epigenetics has shed light on how lifestyle decisions can alter the expression of genes linked to cancer risk in recent years. Epigenetics is the study of how environmental factors, such as nutrition, exercise, & exposure to toxins, can affect gene activity without changing the underlying DNA sequence. Research has indicated that specific lifestyle modifications can alter the expression of genes implicated in the development of cancer, potentially lowering the risk of cancer even in people who are genetically predisposed to it. For example, studies have shown that specific dietary elements, like cruciferous vegetables & folate, can affect the expression of genes linked to cell cycle regulation & DNA repair, which may help prevent cancer. Likewise, it has been demonstrated that exercise influences the expression of genes related to immunological response, inflammation, & tumour growth. This demonstrates how lifestyle decisions have the ability to alter genetic risk factors at the molecular level in addition to lowering the risk of cancer. The idea of personalised medicine, which entails adjusting preventative tactics according to each person's distinct genetic profile, is among the most exciting advancements in cancer prevention. People can now identify particular genetic mutations or risk factors linked to cancer thanks to advancements in genomic sequencing & genetic testing, which empowers them to make better decisions about lifestyle modifications & preventive measures. For instance, people who have a BRCA1 or BRCA2 mutation that makes them genetically predisposed to breast cancer may decide to take chemopreventive drugs like tamoxifen, have more frequent screenings, or alter their diet & level of physical activity. People who are aware of their genetic risks can prevent cancer more actively & individually by adopting lifestyle choices that are best suited to their unique genetic makeup. It's crucial to understand that genetic testing is not deterministic, even though it can yield useful information. Even in the presence of genetic predispositions, a person's lifestyle choices, such as eating a balanced diet, exercising frequently, & abstaining from alcohol & tobacco, can significantly lower their risk of developing cancer. Furthermore, there is still much to learn about the ways that particular lifestyle factors affect cancer risk at the genetic level due to the complex interplay between genes & the environment. There are still many obstacles in the way of encouraging the general adoption of healthy behaviours, even in light of the mounting evidence that links lifestyle choices to the risk of cancer. Genetic counsellors, medical professionals, & public health campaigns are all crucial in informing people about the significance of lifestyle changes in lowering cancer risk, especially for those with genetic predispositions. The main takeaway is that, regardless of one's genetic background, people can take charge of their health & lower their risk of developing cancer by making proactive, educated decisions. To sum up, addressing genetic risks through lifestyle choices provides a potent cancer prevention strategy because it enables people to actively alter their cancer risk profile by adopting habits like eating a balanced diet, exercising frequently, giving up smoking, & consuming less alcohol. Even those with genetic predispositions can lower their risk of developing cancer by combining these lifestyle factors with genetic testing &

personalised cancer screening. Although lifestyle changes cannot completely prevent cancer, they are a significant, scientifically supported strategy for lowering the disease's burden & enhancing general health. The potential for lifestyle decisions to reduce genetic risks will only increase as genomics & personalised medicine research advances, providing people with better ways to prevent cancer & live healthier lives.

The Future Of Cancer Prevention Strategies

Thanks to previously unheard-of developments in technology, personalised medicine, & scientific research, cancer prevention strategies are about to undergo a paradigm shift. As our knowledge of cancer grows, it is becoming more & more obvious that prevention involves using state-of-the-art tools to target the biological mechanisms that underlie the development of cancer, intervene early, & personalise strategies in addition to limiting exposure to known carcinogens. An integrated, multifaceted strategy that incorporates lifestyle changes, genetic & environmental evaluations, early detection technologies, & innovative pharmaceutical interventions to stop cancer before it even starts will define the next era of cancer prevention. The intersection of several scientific disciplines, such as immunology, genomics, epigenetics, & artificial intelligence (AI), which are all changing how we think about cancer risk & prevention, holds the key to this future. The expanding field of genomics, especially in the areas of genetic testing & personalised medicine, is one of the most promising research areas in cancer prevention. The Human Genome Project's completion & continued developments in high-throughput sequencing technologies have made it feasible to detect genetic mutations & predispositions that raise a person's risk of getting cancer. Genetic screening will probably become more common in the future, making it possible to identify high-risk individuals well in advance of the development of cancer. Equipped with this understanding, patients can adopt a proactive preventative strategy, modifying their lifestyle, medical treatments, & surveillance to lower their risk. For instance, people who have inherited mutations in genes like BRCA1 or BRCA2, which are linked to an increased risk of ovarian & breast cancer, might choose to undergo more frequent screenings, have preventive surgery, or take chemopreventive drugs. Furthermore, by incorporating genetic risk assessments into standard medical care, physicians could provide individualised preventative plans based on each patient's distinct genetic profile. By detecting & controlling risks early on, even before malignant changes take place, this strategy may greatly lower the incidence of cancer. The expanding knowledge of the role of epigenetics in the development of cancer is another exciting development for the future of cancer prevention. Changes in gene expression that do not involve changes to the underlying DNA sequence are known as epigenetic modifications, & they are becoming more widely acknowledged as a significant contributor to the development of cancer. Epigenetic changes that either promote or suppress cancer can be influenced by environmental factors, including stress, exposure to toxins, & diet. The prospect of "reprogramming" the epigenome to prevent cancer will become a reality as studies continue to reveal the intricate interactions between genetic & environmental factors. For instance, certain foods, organic substances, & lifestyle changes may be utilised to "turn on" tumor-suppressor genes or "turn off" genes that promote cancer, providing a potent cancer prevention tool. Targeted dietary interventions, exercise routines, & other lifestyle modifications that can alter gene expression & lower the risk of cancer are probably going to be part of this strategy. Immunotherapy is one of the most innovative approaches to cancer prevention. Immunotherapy has demonstrated great promise in the treatment of advanced cancers by using the body's immune system to combat the disease. But in the future, immunotherapy might also be applied as a prophylactic measure, before cancer even appears. Scientists are investigating strategies to encourage the immune system to identify & eradicate precancerous cells or cells with a high propensity to develop into cancer. In order to target particular cancer-associated antigens or markers that are present in the early stages of cancer development, vaccines or other immune-boosting therapies may need to be developed. In this situation, immunotherapy may be a proactive strategy to stop cancer from developing in high-risk individuals or to lower the chance of recurrence in cancer survivors. Future cancer prevention will heavily rely on developments in early detection & diagnostic technologies in addition to immunotherapy. Since cancer is easier to treat & has a better chance of survival the earlier it is discovered, early detection is essential to improving cancer outcomes. Although the incidence & mortality of some cancers have decreased thanks to current screening techniques like Pap smears, colonoscopies, & mammograms, much more needs to be done to increase the sensitivity & specificity of these tests. Highly sensitive, non-invasive screening tests that can identify cancer in its earliest, most treatable stages will be developed in the future of cancer prevention. For instance, liquid biopsy is a promising method that examines blood samples to find tumour DNA, genetic mutations, or other cancer-related biomarkers. Liquid biopsies may eventually be used as standard cancer screening procedures, enabling the early identification of cancers like pancreatic, breast, & lung cancer long before symptoms show up. Furthermore, machine learning & artificial intelligence (AI) algorithms are being incorporated into cancer detection, assisting in the analysis of enormous volumes of data from genetic, imaging, & molecular tests in order to spot trends & make previously unheard-of accurate predictions about cancer risk. Cancer prevention will become more accurate & successful than ever before thanks to the integration of AI, which will enable customised, data-driven prevention strategies based on each person's particular risk profile. The future of cancer prevention will be influenced by advancements in lifestyle interventions, especially in the areas of nutrition, exercise, & environmental exposure, in addition to genetics & early detection. Diet plans that are customised to a person's genetic composition, lifestyle, & health requirements are becoming possible thanks to developments in nutritional science & personalised nutrition. For example, based on a person's genetic predisposition, precision nutrition may make it possible to identify particular dietary patterns or nutrients that can help prevent cancer. Furthermore, studies on the gut microbiota—an ecosystem of microorganisms that reside in & on our bodies—have shown that it is essential for preserving immunological function & averting illness, including cancer. With targeted probiotics, prebiotics, & dietary changes intended to improve gut health & lower cancer risk, personalised microbiome interventions may one day play a significant role in cancer prevention. A key component of cancer prevention will remain physical activity, as there is mounting evidence that regular exercise lowers the risk of developing a number of cancers. Exercise plans customised for each person based on their genetic & epigenetic profiles are expected to be developed in the future as research in this area advances, maximising the benefits of physical activity in preventing cancer. Future initiatives to prevent cancer will also concentrate on environmental exposures, including pollution, hazardous chemicals, & UV radiation. Innovative public health programs & policies targeted at lowering exposure to environmental carcinogens will be crucial in preventing cancer at the population level, even though environmental factors are mostly out of an individual's control. Furthermore, developments in environmental health research will keep revealing fresh strategies to lessen the effects of dangerous exposures, like creating safer chemicals, enhancing workplace safety, & launching more successful public health initiatives. In addition to lowering risk factors, the future of cancer prevention will prioritise individualised risk management strategies. Cancer prevention will become more customised, focused, & efficient by utilising developments in genetic testing, early detection, immunotherapy, lifestyle modifications, & environmental health. A proactive, preventive model of cancer treatment, where most cancers are stopped before they even have a chance to develop, will eventually replace the current reactive approach. Even though there is still a lot of work to be done, the future of cancer prevention is bright, with hope for a world where people are empowered to take charge of their health & cancer incidence & mortality are drastically decreased. Future cancer prevention techniques have the potential to transform healthcare, enhance quality of life, & lessen the global cancer burden with sustained investment in research, technology, & education.

CHAPTER 6: CRAFTING YOUR PERSONALIZED PREVENTION PLAN.

One of the most effective & empowering strategies to lower your risk of developing cancer while enhancing your general health & well-being is to create a customised cancer prevention plan. This method goes beyond general guidelines by concentrating on each person's distinct genetic composition, way of life, exposures to the environment, & personal health objectives in order to develop a customised plan that takes into account their needs, preferences, & risks. A comprehensive evaluation of risk factors, such as genetic predispositions, lifestyle choices, environmental factors, & family history, is the first step in developing a personalised cancer prevention plan. This is followed by the creation of practical measures to reduce those risks. Knowing your genetic risk is the first important step in creating a customised prevention strategy. People can now have their DNA examined to find particular genetic mutations or markers linked to a higher risk of developing certain cancers thanks to the development of genetic testing technologies. For instance, people with Lynch syndrome may be more susceptible to colorectal, endometrial, or other cancers, while those with mutations in the BRCA1 or BRCA2 genes may be much more likely to develop breast or ovarian cancer. People can better understand their own risk profile through genetic testing, which gives them the chance to take preventative actions like more screenings, preventive drugs, or even surgery, depending on the level of risk found. Apart from genetic factors, lifestyle choices are crucial in preventing cancer, & lowering overall risk requires addressing these factors. Adopting a healthy diet is one of the most effective lifestyle modifications for preventing cancer. Essential nutrients, antioxidants, & fibre that support the body's natural defences & help prevent cancer can be found in a diet high in fruits, vegetables, whole grains, lean proteins, & healthy fats. Antioxidants, like vitamins C & E, which are present in fruits & vegetables, for instance, aid in scavenging dangerous free radicals that can cause cell damage & cancer. Plant-based foods contain fibre, which is essential for preserving digestive health & averting colorectal cancer. It's also critical to cut back on processed foods, red meat, & sugary drinks because these foods have been connected to an increased risk of developing a number of cancers. You can make long-lasting, sustainable changes that will lower your risk of cancer & enhance your general health by customising your diet to fit your lifestyle, cultural preferences, & personal health objectives. Physical activity is another essential lifestyle component in preventing cancer. Frequent exercise has been demonstrated to reduce the risk of endometrial, colon, & breast cancer, among other cancers. Exercise aids in the regulation of hormones like insulin & oestrogen, which are associated with the development of cancer when they are present in excess. Additionally, it lowers inflammation, boosts the immune system, & aids in maintaining a healthy weight—all of which help prevent cancer. Finding an enjoyable &

sustainable exercise routine is crucial, whether that be strength training, yoga, cycling, swimming, or walking. A general recommendation for enhancing cancer prevention is to include two or more days of strength training in addition to at least 150 minutes of moderate-intensity aerobic activity per week. A customised exercise program can help maximise the cancer-preventive benefits of physical activity for people with particular genetic predispositions. Because obesity is a major risk factor for a number of cancers, including breast, colon, & pancreatic cancer, maintaining a healthy weight is another crucial component of a cancer prevention strategy. A healthy weight must be attained & maintained through diet & exercise because excess body fat generates hormones & inflammatory molecules that can encourage the growth of cancer. Making small, sustainable changes that fit your lifestyle is crucial if controlling your weight is a top priority in your prevention strategy. Environmental exposures are just as important in preventing cancer as genetic & lifestyle factors. Reducing cancer risk requires an understanding of & commitment to minimising exposure to environmental toxins, pollutants, & carcinogens. For instance, the risk of lung cancer, skin cancer, & other cancers can be decreased by limiting exposure to tobacco smoke, air pollution, & specific chemicals found in household products. Skin cancer risk can also be considerably decreased by practicing sun safety, which includes wearing sunscreen, protective clothes, & finding shade. This is especially important for people with fair skin or a family history of skin cancer.

Avoiding known carcinogens is even more crucial in certain situations where people with a high genetic risk for a particular cancer may be especially susceptible to environmental exposures. People must also take mental & emotional health into consideration when creating a truly customised cancer prevention plan. Chronic stress, anxiety, & depression can significantly affect one's general health & may be linked to the development of cancer through immune suppression, inflammation, & hormone imbalances, among other mechanisms. It is possible to manage stress & foster a sense of peace & wellbeing by engaging in stress-reduction practices like yoga, meditation, deep breathing exercises, & mindfulness. Additionally, getting help from support groups or mental health specialists can offer helpful strategies for managing stress & enhancing resilience. Better mental health & better health outcomes can also result from adopting a positive outlook on life & partaking in mental wellness-promoting activities like hobbies, spending time with loved ones, & practicing gratitude. A mix of the above-mentioned tactics will probably be used in the future of personalised cancer prevention, incorporated into a coherent & flexible strategy that changes as new knowledge, tools, & research become available. For instance, improvements in genomics & personalised medicine will enable even more accurate recommendations based on a person's lifestyle choices, genetic composition, & epigenetic profile. Future cancer prevention strategies may incorporate probiotic interventions & customised nutrition aimed at promoting gut health & lowering inflammation as knowledge about the gut microbiota & its connection to cancer prevention continues to expand. Because AI & machine learning can analyse large amounts of data from genetic testing, medical histories, & lifestyle factors to find patterns & predict cancer risk, they will also be used in personalised cancer prevention. Healthcare professionals will be able to develop highly customised prevention plans that cater to each patient's unique needs with the aid of AI, offering the most efficient & scientifically supported methods for lowering the risk of cancer. Additionally, by giving people real-time feedback on their stress levels, sleep patterns, exercise routines, & diet, wearable technology & health tracking applications will enable people to take charge of their health. These resources can be incorporated into individualised prevention programs, assisting people in maintaining their health objectives & making necessary modifications. Regarding medical interventions, targeted chemoprevention strategies for high-risk individuals may also be developed in the future. Supplements or medications that reduce the risk of cancer may be included in individualised prevention programs for people with particular risk factors or genetic mutations. For instance, people who are at a high risk of breast cancer might be prescribed drugs like aromatase inhibitors or tamoxifen to lower their chance of getting the disease. Aspirin or other anti-inflammatory drugs may also be helpful for people who have a genetic predisposition to colorectal cancer as part of their preventative strategy. Advances in immunotherapy could lead to vaccines or other immune-boosting treatments that can stop cancer before it starts, in addition to medical interventions. Preventive immunotherapies that target precancerous cells or genetic mutations linked to cancer may be developed as a result of future research, as immunotherapy has already demonstrated success in treating cancers that are already present. These treatments could be combined with early detection techniques & lifestyle changes to provide a thorough, multifaceted approach to cancer prevention. Finally, it is critical to understand that a customised cancer prevention plan should change over time in response to shifts in a person's health, risk factors, & new scientific findings rather than being a static or one-time procedure. To track progress, reevaluate risks, & modify the prevention strategy as necessary, routine follow-up with medical professionals, genetic counsellors, & other experts is crucial. This could entail introducing new screening technologies, revising lifestyle advice, updating genetic tests, or investigating novel pharmacological treatments. A sustained dedication to proactive health management & a readiness to adapt as new information becomes available are essential components of a successful personalised prevention plan. In summary, developing a personalised cancer prevention plan is a highly customised process that considers lifestyle, genetic, environmental, & emotional factors to develop a customised approach to cancer risk reduction. You can greatly lower your risk of getting cancer & enhance your general health by being aware of your particular risk factors & taking proactive measures to change them. Personalised, evidence-based strategies that combine state-of-the-art research, technology, & medical interventions to offer the most efficient & focused approaches for every individual are the way of the future for cancer prevention. People will be able to take charge of their health & collaborate with medical professionals to develop a dynamic & changing cancer prevention plan that maximises their health outcomes through a combination of genetic testing, lifestyle changes, early detection, & new therapies. People can lower their risk of developing cancer, increase longevity, & ultimately lead healthier, more satisfying lives if they have the appropriate resources, information, & support.

Setting Goals For A Healthier Lifestyle

Establishing objectives for a healthier lifestyle is a potent & life-changing process that calls for careful consideration, dedication, & strategic preparation. The quest for improved health necessitates a holistic strategy that takes into account different facets of mental, emotional, & physical well-being, with each component cooperating to produce long-lasting, sustainable effects. Determining what health means to you personally is the first step in creating goals for a healthier lifestyle. A multifaceted concept, health includes mental clarity, emotional stability, physical fitness, dietary practices, & general life satisfaction. A person's needs, obstacles, priorities, & objectives can all greatly influence what they consider to be a healthier lifestyle. Since health is a unique journey that changes over time rather than a one-size-fits-all undertaking, it is crucial to approach goal-setting with adaptability & an open mind. Setting SMART (specific, measurable, achievable, relevant, & time-bound) goals is the next step after you have a clear idea of what health means to you. This framework is essential because it gives you focus & clarity, which guarantees that your objectives are reasonable & in line with your long-term health vision. A SMART goal might be, for instance, to work out for 30 minutes five days a week for the next three months. This objective is time-bound (set for the next three months), relevant (important for general health), measurable (five days a week), achievable (a reasonable amount of exercise), & specific (exercise for 30 minutes). Establishing SMART goals makes it simpler to stay on course & track progress by breaking down more complex objectives into smaller, more manageable steps. Understanding that health is a dynamic, continuous process & that consistency & dedication are necessary to achieve long-lasting results is another essential element of creating health goals. Setting lofty, short-term objectives that promise quick results is alluring, but it's crucial to concentrate on long-term sustainability. For instance, think about establishing a more sustainable goal of losing 1-2 pounds every week for the next six months, as opposed to aiming to lose 10 pounds in a month. Instead of an unsustainable crash diet that could result in yo-yo dieting & detrimental health effects, this method enables gradual, sustainable weight loss that can be sustained over time. Similar to this, when it comes to exercise, instead of committing to rigorous sessions every day, think about establishing a goal to create a regular routine by beginning with achievable objectives & progressively increasing the length or intensity of your sessions as your level of fitness increases. Building enduring habits requires consistency, & you have a better chance of succeeding & gaining momentum over time if you set attainable goals. A comprehensive approach to goal-setting that addresses various facets of health & wellbeing is also crucial. Even though physical health is frequently the main priority, mental & emotional health are just as crucial to general health. Goals for mental health can include techniques that help people focus better, feel less stressed, & become more emotionally resilient, like journaling, mindfulness, meditation, or therapy. Establishing objectives for bettering mental health could entail making a commitment to meditation every day, going to therapy sessions on a regular basis, or taking breaks during the day to recover & rejuvenate. Since long-term stress & negative emotions can have a significant impact on physical health & contribute to conditions like heart disease, obesity, & compromised immune function, emotional well-being is just as important as physical fitness. You can develop a more integrated & balanced approach to health by integrating mental & emotional health objectives into your overall lifestyle plan. Prioritising flexibility & self-compassion is another crucial component of creating goals for a healthier lifestyle. Because life is unpredictable, challenges, setbacks, & obstacles are inevitable. It's critical to understand that leading a healthier lifestyle is about progress rather than perfection. Accept the notion that obstacles are a normal aspect of the process & ought to be seen as teaching moments rather than as failures. For instance, refrain from feeling guilty or critical of yourself if you skip a workout or overindulge in unhealthy foods during a holiday celebration. Rather, accept the loss, consider how you can change your strategy going forward, & reaffirm your commitment to your objectives. Developing self-compassion helps you avoid burnout or demotivation & keeps you resilient & driven even in the face of adversity. Similarly, since priorities, health, & life circumstances can change over time, it's critical to be flexible with your goals. For instance, your exercise objectives might need to be modified to account for your recuperation if you are recovering from an injury. You can keep feeling like you're making progress without getting frustrated by unanticipated setbacks if you're adaptable & adjust your goals to your current circumstances. Tracking & evaluating your progress is another essential component of creating goals for a healthier lifestyle. You can stay accountable, evaluate your accomplishments, & pinpoint areas for improvement by keeping track of your health-related objectives. Tracking can be done in a variety of ways, such as keeping a journal or using smartphone apps to keep tabs on your food, exercise, sleep, & mental health, or just regularly checking in with yourself to see how you're feeling emotionally & physically. You can make better decisions about your health & modify your goals as necessary by routinely assessing your progress & spotting trends & patterns.

For instance, you might decide to establish a bedtime routine or cut back on screen time before bed if you find that you're constantly having trouble getting enough sleep. In addition to keeping you inspired, tracking your progress enables you to stay focused on your objectives & make any necessary adjustments to guarantee success. The significance of social networks & support networks in attaining a healthier lifestyle is a crucial goal-setting component that is frequently disregarded. Your chances of success can be greatly increased by having a strong support system, whether it be made up of friends, family, coworkers, or online communities. Support networks offer motivation, accountability, & encouragement, particularly in the face of difficulties or periods of uncertainty. Joining a fitness group or working out with a friend, for instance, can help you stick to your goals & make exercise more fun. Similar to this, having a friend or relative who has similar health objectives to your own can help you stay on track & reinforce healthy habits if you're trying to improve your diet. Additionally, social ties are important for mental & emotional health. Stress can be decreased, mood can be lifted, & feelings of contentment & happiness can be increased by spending time with loved ones, exchanging stories, & having deep conversations. Creating a support network that complements your health objectives can help you stay motivated & make the process more pleasurable & long-lasting. Last but not least, recognising the value of balance is necessary to establish reasonable goals for a healthier lifestyle. It's crucial to concentrate on improving your diet, exercise routine, & general health, but it's also critical to keep a healthy balance & refrain from taking on too much at once. Burnout can result from attempting to make all the changes at once. Instead, concentrate on one or two important areas at a time, & as you gain momentum & confidence, progressively broaden your goals. For instance, if increasing your level of fitness is your main objective, start by concentrating on developing a regular exercise schedule. You can start incorporating other objectives, like bettering your diet or sleeping patterns, once you are at ease with your exercise routine. A balanced, methodical approach will increase your chances of long-term success & keep you from becoming overwhelmed by irrational expectations. To sum up, establishing objectives for a healthier lifestyle is a very personal & life-changing process that entails determining your own needs, priorities, & values before creating a methodical, doable plan to reach them. You can make sure your health goals are clear, attainable, & realistic by using the SMART framework to set specific, measurable, achievable, relevant, & time-bound goals. Achieving your goals also involves taking into account your mental & emotional well-being, putting self-compassion & adaptability first, monitoring your progress, asking for help when you need it, & keeping a healthy balance. Keep in mind that adopting a healthier lifestyle is a continuous process that calls for perseverance, patience, & dedication. You can make long-lasting, beneficial changes that will raise your quality of life & improve your general well-being by making tiny, regular progress towards your health objectives & modifying your strategy as necessary. You can attain the healthier lifestyle you want with perseverance, self-compassion, & a clear sense of purpose. Progress, not perfection, is the key to success.

Tracking Progress & Staying Motivated

When it comes to personal goals, especially those related to health & wellness, tracking progress & maintaining motivation are essential components of reaching & sustaining long-term success. Both of these elements are necessary to guarantee that people stay on course, keep going, & eventually achieve their intended results. Despite its apparent simplicity, progress tracking is frequently disregarded or underutilised, despite being one of the most effective strategies for success. Keeping a detailed journal, using apps or devices that measure important metrics like physical activity, food intake, sleep, & even emotional well-being, or creating goal charts or visual reminders that offer immediate feedback are just a few of the many ways that tracking can be done. While each of these tracking techniques has advantages of its own, they all aim to provide the person with concrete proof of their journey. When it comes to health-related objectives, especially long-term ones, it's simple to lose motivation when setbacks or slow progress appear. Tracking serves as a reminder of your progress by offering a quantitative & qualitative record of your efforts. For instance, if your objective is to get more fit or lose weight, it can be very inspiring to watch your weight gradually drop or your endurance grow over time. Tracking also enables you to recognise & appreciate minor accomplishments, like a week of regular exercise or eating a healthy diet, which can help you feel more accomplished. When these minor victories are recognised & celebrated, they serve as a source of ongoing inspiration & give you the drive to keep going despite obstacles. Additionally, tracking identifies areas that might require modification. Examining your logs, for example, can assist you in identifying possible areas of concern if you're not seeing the desired results. For example, you might be getting insufficient sleep or your exercise regimen may not be as consistent as you initially believed. You can make sure your efforts are as successful as possible by keeping a thorough record of your progress, which gives you the chance to reflect & adjust your strategy as needed. But tracking by itself is insufficient. Long-term dedication to wellness & health objectives requires constant nurturing of motivation, a complex & multidimensional force. Motivation is subject to change & frequently depends on both internal & external factors. When you are motivated by internal factors, such as happiness, fulfilment, or personal development, you act on it. Conversely, extrinsic motivation is fuelled by outside incentives or pressures, like the need to attain a particular body image or receive a reward for accomplishing a goal. While both forms of motivation are important, intrinsic motivation is typically more effective for long-term success. Linking your health objectives to a more profound sense of meaning or purpose is crucial for developing intrinsic motivation. For instance, concentrating on how better nutrition or exercise increases your energy, elevates your mood, or improves your general quality of life can be far more motivating than concentrating only on achieving purely aesthetic objectives, like dropping pounds or getting into a particular size. Finding the "why" behind your health objectives is one of the best strategies to maintain motivation because it makes the process more emotionally engaging & guarantees that your objectives are consistent with your values. Visualising your success is another strategy to keep yourself motivated. You can strengthen your commitment to your goals by visualising yourself reaching your health goals or envisioning the positive effects it will have on your life. Visualisation is a powerful technique that has been used by successful people in a variety of fields, including athletes & performers. When it comes to health & well-being, visualisation can increase self-assurance, lower anxiety, & motivate people to keep moving forward. This is especially beneficial when obstacles appear or motivation starts to decline. Your drive can be greatly increased by outside sources of support in addition to internal motivation. Having a support network is crucial for many people to stay motivated. Having someone to hold you accountable, offer support, or share the journey with can greatly improve your chances of success, whether that person is a friend who keeps track of your progress, a workout partner, or a community group with like-minded objectives. Incentives, acknowledgement, or positive reinforcement are further ways that support can manifest. No matter how big or small your milestones are, it's important to celebrate them in ways that are meaningful to you. This could be as easy as giving yourself a treat, like a small indulgence, a favourite meal, or a restful day off, or it could be as complex as publicly recognising your progress by telling friends or followers on social media about your accomplishments. These outside motivators support your dedication to the goal by giving you a sense of accomplishment & acknowledgement. But when it comes to motivation, it's important to keep a balanced viewpoint. Variations in your motivation & energy levels are common, especially when working towards long-term objectives. Sometimes motivation will be strong, & other times it will seem elusive. In times of low energy, it's critical to rely on the mechanisms you've established, such as monitoring your progress, getting motivation from your support system, & re-establishing your connection to your inner "why." Additionally, it can be simpler to persevere through challenging times if you have a growth mindset, which holds that obstacles are chances for learning & development. Adopt a mindset that sees challenges & setbacks as essential components of the journey, required for fostering resilience & personal development, rather than as failures. It's also important to remember that motivation isn't always centred around big gestures or noteworthy accomplishments. Focussing on consistency rather than perfection can occasionally be the most effective strategy for maintaining motivation. Little daily activities, like exercising a little, choosing nutritious foods, or setting aside some time for meditation, can add up over time to form enduring habits. Maintaining your commitment to your bigger goals can be made easier by keeping track of these little victories on a daily basis. Adapting your goals as necessary is another essential component of maintaining motivation. Your priorities & circumstances change as life does. It's acceptable to change your goals to better suit your needs if you discover that a particular one no longer feels relevant or if your lifestyle or health condition changes. For instance, your emphasis may change from intense workouts to softer activities like stretching or swimming if you're recuperating from an injury. Being able to adjust to changing conditions & maintain your flexibility will prevent you from losing hope or giving up on your objectives completely. Additionally, it keeps you from feeling like a failure if you are unable to meet a deadline or goal. You can continue to move forward in a sustainable & useful manner by modifying your goals to fit your life. Furthermore, the power of habits is closely linked to motivation & tracking. The development of healthy habits that eventually become second nature is frequently what propels long-lasting progress. When intentionally formed, these behaviours support advancement with less mental strain. For example, planning your workouts for the same time every day or cooking nutritious meals ahead of time can help you stay on track without having to remind yourself all the time. As habits become engrained in your daily routine, tracking your progress helps reinforce them. Habits are like the scaffolding that supports long-term change. According to the adage, "what gets measured gets improved." Making tracking a regular component of your procedure generates a continuous feedback loop that motivates you to keep going & promotes improvement. Finally, it's critical to recognise that maintaining motivation & monitoring progress are ongoing processes. Both motivation & progress are dynamic. Both fluctuate, & that's acceptable. The secret is to create routines that help you stay focused on your objectives even on days when you don't feel motivated. While keeping an eye on intrinsic motivation guarantees that the journey stays meaningful, tracking also helps provide objective data that can validate your efforts. No matter what obstacles you face, you can stay on track, adjust to them, & keep working towards your wellness & health objectives if you have the correct tools, techniques, & attitude.

Overcoming Setbacks & Roadblocks

Reaching long-term goals requires overcoming obstacles & setbacks, especially when attempting to improve oneself or reach wellness, fitness, or health goals. No path to success is ever free of obstacles, & retaining resilience, adaptability, & focus requires an awareness that setbacks are an unavoidable aspect of the process. Recognising & accepting setbacks instead of seeing them as failures or insurmountable obstacles is the first step towards conquering them. Life is full of setbacks, & how we handle them often determines whether we advance or get caught in a vicious cycle of frustration & self-doubt. For example, it's critical to understand that a person's journey isn't defined by these moments if their goal is to lose weight but they instead experience a period of stagnation or gain weight. Rather, failures ought to be seen as chances for introspection & education. When setbacks happen, it's usually because we've faced unforeseen obstacles, whether they be internal (like a lack of drive, self-doubt, or negative emotions) or external (like a hectic schedule, illness, or environmental factors). The first step in either scenario is to fight the impulse to give up completely or to become discouraged. Taking a step back & conducting an unbiased analysis of the situation can yield important insights into the reasons behind the setback. For instance, poor time management or irrational expectations may be the reason behind a person's inability to maintain consistency in their exercise regimen. A more effective response is possible when the underlying cause of the setback is understood. Making a plan for the future is the next step after determining the cause. To get past the obstacle, this plan may entail modifying objectives, schedules, or tactics. For example, rather than trying to do too much at once, someone who is feeling overwhelmed by their workout regimen might choose to gradually increase the length or intensity of their exercises. As an alternative, they might decide to reallocate time for physical activity in a way that better suits their lifestyle after realising that their current workout routine is unsustainable. It's critical to address the psychological elements causing setbacks when they are brought on by internal obstacles like emotional difficulties, negative self-talk, or a lack of motivation. When faced with obstacles, people frequently give up on their goals completely due to self-doubt or a fear of failing. Developing a resilient & self-compassionate mindset is essential in these situations. People should be patient & kind to themselves instead of criticising themselves for not getting the results they want. This could entail changing pessimistic ideas into more positive ones, like acknowledging that failures are common & that development is not always linear. People can lessen the psychological impact of setbacks & regain the drive to keep going forward by accepting that they are transient & a normal part of the goal-setting process. The ability to be flexible & adaptable is another essential component in conquering obstacles. It is crucial to understand that plans & goals should be adaptable enough to change with the times rather than being inflexible. Due to the unpredictability of life, plans may need to be modified when circumstances arise. For instance, if someone is injured while attempting to run a marathon, this setback might necessitate a short-term change in strategy. The person may change their objective to prioritise recovery over pushing through the injury & running the risk of more damage, then progressively resume training as soon as they are physically capable. Here, flexibility respects the body's need for rest & recuperation while enabling the person to maintain alignment with their long-term health objectives. Setbacks can be transformed into growth opportunities by modifying the schedule or strategy, as people gain the ability to overcome obstacles with greater consideration & knowledge. Another important element in overcoming obstacles is surrounding oneself with support networks. Overcoming obstacles alone can be challenging, especially when we're feeling overburdened or alone. In times of adversity, having a solid support system—whether it be friends, family, a coach, a therapist, or an online community—can offer accountability, inspiration, & encouragement. When obstacles arise, discussing them with others enables a fresh viewpoint & frequently provides answers or concepts that might not have been thought of. Additionally, by reminding people of their accomplishments, a support system can help them see beyond the short-term setbacks in their journey. Furthermore, receiving support from others can boost morale in moments of frustration or uncertainty by offering emotional encouragement. For instance, if someone is feeling depressed about their progress towards weight loss, a friend who is encouraging might remind them of their accomplishments or motivate them to continue by sharing a workout experience or motivation. The capacity to maintain focus on the long-term goal rather than becoming overwhelmed by short-term setbacks or frustrations is another crucial component of overcoming setbacks. Setbacks can frequently feel like a huge blow when working towards a bigger goal, like reaching a fitness milestone or improving general health, especially when progress seems to slow down or plateau. Nonetheless, people can continue to be dedicated to the journey by considering the long-term advantages. Reminding oneself of the initial significance of the goal is crucial. To stay focused on the big picture, someone who is trying to get healthier might, for instance, keep a visual reminder of their objective, like a picture, an inspirational saying, or a health journal. This long-term view enables people to stay focused on the goal even in the face of adversity & keeps setbacks from feeling overwhelming. Furthermore, it may be simpler to overcome obstacles if more ambitious objectives are divided into smaller, more doable steps. Big, long-term objectives can frequently seem overwhelming, & failures can make them appear even farther off. Even in the face of setbacks, people can make consistent progress by segmenting their goals into smaller, incremental milestones. Even though the bigger goal is still a work in progress, these smaller steps also make it easier to track progress, which can inspire motivation & a sense of accomplishment. If someone wants to lose fifty pounds, for instance, breaking that down into weekly weight-loss milestones or monthly targets can help them feel like they're making progress & that the goal is more reachable. People can modify their strategy or timetable in response to setbacks, but they should continue to concentrate on these incremental victories. The power of persistence is another useful tactic for conquering obstacles. The capacity to keep going after objectives in the face of difficulties or obstacles is known as persistence. Having a mindset that sees setbacks as temporary & as chances to improve is essential to cultivating persistence. It's critical to keep in mind that setbacks are a necessary component of learning & not a sign of failure. Even when things seem challenging or progress is slow, persistence enables people to remain dedicated to their objectives. This change in perspective can be immensely empowering because it enables people to view obstacles as opportunities to reach their ultimate goals rather than as insurmountable obstacles. The knowledge that results take time is another factor that fuels persistence. Real progress is frequently gradual & necessitates consistent effort over time, despite the temptation to want results right away in a world of instant gratification. People can maintain their resilience & motivation by realising this & accepting that failures are a natural part of the process. Last but not least, taking care of oneself & striking a healthy balance between work & relaxation are two of the most crucial tactics for conquering obstacles. Setbacks can occasionally be an indication that the body or mind needs a rest. Burnout & additional setbacks can result from overworking oneself, ignoring the need for rest, or pushing through fatigue. It's critical to pay attention to your body's signals & allow yourself to take breaks when necessary. Maintaining the energy & fortitude required to overcome obstacles requires taking care of one's physical & mental well-being through routines like meditation, adequate sleep, stress reduction, & a healthy diet. Progress requires rest & recuperation, & by making self-care a priority, people can develop the endurance required to keep going. In summary, conquering obstacles & setbacks is a crucial component of any personal growth process, particularly when aiming for wellness, fitness, or health objectives.

Reframing setbacks as learning opportunities, modifying tactics, & keeping a long-term outlook are the keys to overcoming them. Despite obstacles, people can keep going by acknowledging setbacks as a normal part of the process, figuring out what caused them, & modifying their plans or goals. Overcoming setbacks requires a combination of resilience, self-compassion, support networks, & flexibility. By maintaining perspective, people can transform setbacks into opportunities. With the correct attitude, tactics, & dedication to advancement, setbacks don't have to define the path; rather, they can be potent stimulants for development & change.

Building A Support Network For Lasting Change

One of the most effective strategies for attaining personal transformation & maintaining long-term advancement in any area of life—be it relationships, career, health, fitness, or general personal development—is creating a support system for long-lasting change. Achieving long-lasting change can be a difficult journey, & going it alone frequently results in feelings of failure, frustration, & loneliness. People can stay on course, overcome challenges, & maintain motivation throughout their journey with the emotional, social, & practical resources that a robust, well-rounded support network offers. Understanding the kind of support required & realising that no one person can provide all facets of that support is the first step in creating an effective support network. Finding people who can provide a mix of support, accountability, direction, & empathy based on one's individual objectives is necessary when building a network. First & foremost, when attempting to bring about long-lasting change, emotional support is frequently the most important element. Change can be a challenging & emotionally draining process, especially when it entails forming new routines or kicking old habits. The emotional load is lessened when there are people who can listen, understand, & sympathise when difficulties occur. Family members, close friends, or even support groups that are aware of the particular difficulties being faced can provide emotional support. These individuals act as a sounding board, offering confirmation & assurance that difficulties & setbacks are typical aspects of the process & do not signify failure. People who receive emotional support feel less alone, & the inspiration they receive during trying times can give them the willpower to keep going. Accountability is another essential component of a support system. Accountability partners are people who monitor progress, assist in establishing reasonable objectives, & make sure that promises are kept. Accountability is frequently the key to avoiding procrastination, remaining disciplined, & sustaining focus when it comes to bringing about long-term change. Without someone to hold you accountable, it is simple to veer off course, but having someone to report your progress to & share your goals with fosters a sense of accountability. A coach, mentor, or expert in your field could be your accountability partner, or it could be a friend or relative who helps you keep your word. For instance, having a workout partner who joins them for sessions or a nutritionist who follows up on their dietary choices can help someone stay motivated & on track when they are working towards a health-related goal. Accountability also encourages teamwork & a sense of shared effort. Reporting progress to another person helps to maintain motivation & engagement over time by reinforcing the value of consistency & follow-through. In addition to keeping people on track, a good accountability partner offers helpful criticism, acknowledges accomplishments, & assists in resolving issues when they come up. This mutually beneficial relationship strengthens dedication to the objective & fosters a cooperative environment that may make pursuing long-term change seem more doable. In addition to emotional support & accountability, a strong support network must include mentorship & guidance, particularly when the changes being sought call for new abilities, know-how, or experience. A mentor is a person with experience or knowledge in the field being changed, & they can offer insightful counsel, helpful tips, & doable tactics for success. Mentors can assist in defining the future, providing tried-&-true methods for conquering challenges, & assisting people in avoiding typical pitfalls. A mentor in the desired field could be helpful to someone looking to change careers, a nutritionist or fitness expert could be helpful to someone trying to adopt a healthier lifestyle, or a therapist or counsellor could be helpful to someone trying to improve their personal relationships. The responsibilities of a mentor include guiding when confusion or uncertainty arises, offering advice based on personal experience, & promoting development & progress. Their capacity to mentor & impart knowledge speeds up the transformation process & assists people in avoiding needless setbacks. Apart from mentors, communities or groups with similar objectives can also provide guidance. Whether they are online or in person, these communities can promote a feeling of community & provide collective wisdom. For instance, support groups are extremely helpful for people going through major life transitions like addiction recovery, grieving, or changing their lifestyle. Sharing experiences with people who are going through similar things fosters camaraderie & offers a forum for learning from the triumphs & setbacks of others. Being a part of a community that provides helpful guidance, pooled resources, & compassionate support can help people feel less alone & more understood on their journey. Furthermore, people must actively participate in their network & foster mutually beneficial relationships if they want to create a support system for long-lasting change. Strong support networks are created via mutual care, work, & investment rather than being created in a vacuum. Providing assistance to others, whether through active engagement, advice, or encouragement, fortifies the network & fosters a sense of community. Giving back to one's support system strengthens bonds within the group & fosters a culture of cooperation, trust, & mutual success. In many respects, helping others along the way strengthens one's own sense of purpose & dedication to one's own objectives. Giving advice to someone else who is attempting to change their habits, for example, not only helps the other person but also strengthens the person's own resolve to achieve their wellness objectives. Support-giving & -receiving generates a positive feedback loop that fortifies the network & advances the objectives of all parties. The inclusion of a range of viewpoints & voices is another essential component of a robust support system. Creating a network with a diverse group of people, each with their own experiences & methods, can yield a wider range of success strategies & insights. By exposing people to various perspectives & approaches to problem-solving, diversity promotes resilience, creativity, & innovation. For instance, someone pursuing personal development or transformation may find it helpful to get guidance or inspiration from others with diverse experiences, backgrounds, or fields of expertise. These varied viewpoints question accepted wisdom & expose people to fresh concepts, which can be essential for getting past obstacles & figuring out different ways to proceed when faced with challenges. Additionally, developing a varied support system promotes flexibility, acceptance, & openness—all of which are essential for long-term success & change. Making sure that a strong support network is based on mutual respect & trust is another important component. Any meaningful relationship must be built on trust, which is especially crucial in support groups where members are sharing sensitive details about their lives, like hardships, fears, or failures. Being open, truthful, & judgment-free while offering support is essential to fostering trust within the network. People are more inclined to be honest about their struggles & advancements when they have faith in their support network, which fosters deeper connections & increased responsibility. Furthermore, trust enables people to be open & honest about their true emotions because they know that they will be received with empathy, understanding, & constructive support rather than criticism. Respect-building within the network is equally important. Respect for one another's beliefs, limits, & life experiences creates a mutually understanding atmosphere where people are at ease asking for & giving support. This respectful & trusting culture makes it safe for people to grow as individuals & encourages the formation of deep, enduring bonds. Practical support in the form of shared resources, tools, or logistical assistance can also be essential for overcoming obstacles & maintaining long-term change, even though the significance of emotional support, accountability, guidance, & trust cannot be overstated. In order to make more room for change, practical support could include aiding with time management, offering resources like exercise gear or educational materials, or helping with everyday chores. For instance, if someone is attempting to improve their nutrition & diet, a friend or family member could assist them with meal preparation, grocery shopping, or even cooking classes. People can concentrate more on the larger picture when they offer practical support, which helps to alleviate some of the logistical obstacles that frequently impede progress. Furthermore, because it reaffirms that change is achievable & worthwhile, practical support can be immensely inspiring. One that is flexible & changes with time is a support system for long-lasting change. People's support needs may change as they move through various phases of change. A robust network continues to be flexible, providing the required instruments, materials, & support throughout the process. A strong support network remains a vital resource, offering continuous direction, motivation, & accountability, whether a person is embarking on a journey of transformation, overcoming obstacles, or commemorating achievements. Lastly, it's critical to recognise that no one person or organisation can offer all the assistance required for success. Establishing a varied support system that consists of peers, mentors, professionals, & loved ones is essential to establishing a long-lasting system. A strong, encouraging network increases the chances of overcoming obstacles & accomplishing goals, even though the path to long-lasting change may involve facing difficulties & setbacks. A comprehensive support system offers the motivation, responsibility, tools, & viewpoints required to promote long-lasting change, making the transformation process seem more doable, rewarding, & long-lasting.

Your Action Plan For Long-Term Cancer Prevention

A comprehensive strategy that incorporates a range of lifestyle decisions, routines, & behaviours that together lower the risk of cancer while enhancing general health & well-being is necessary when developing an action plan for long-term cancer prevention. It is impossible to overestimate the significance of a comprehensive, customised action plan because cancer prevention is a complex process that includes proactive steps to lower genetic, environmental, & lifestyle risk factors in addition to encouraging a positive outlook & dedication to continuous health care. Assessing one's current lifestyle & identifying potential risk factors, such as eating patterns, physical activity levels, exposure to environmental pollutants, & medical history, is the first step in creating such a plan. Adopting a healthy & balanced diet that emphasises nutrient-dense, whole foods while minimising processed foods, refined sugars, & unhealthy fats is the first crucial component of the action plan after this assessment. Given that some foods have been demonstrated to have anti-cancer qualities & others may promote the growth of cancerous cells, diet is a critical factor in preventing cancer. Consuming a range of fruits, vegetables, whole grains, legumes, & healthy fats such as those in nuts, seeds, & olive oil can help the body fight off cancer by lowering inflammation & boosting the immune system. A lower risk of several cancers has also been associated with eating foods high in antioxidants, vitamins, & minerals, such as leafy greens, berries, cruciferous vegetables like broccoli & cauliflower, & foods high in fibre. Avoiding excessive alcohol consumption, which has been linked to an increased risk of cancers like breast, liver, & oral cancers, & limiting the consumption of red & processed meats, which have been linked to an increased risk of colorectal & other cancers, are also crucial. Since overeating & unhealthful weight gain are risk factors that can increase the chance of developing cancer, portion control & moderation are important concepts to incorporate into a long-term cancer prevention strategy. Regular exercise is another essential component of cancer prevention, in addition to diet. Exercise not only lowers the risk of obesity-related cancers by helping people maintain a healthy weight, but it also enhances the body's capacity to control hormones like oestrogen & insulin, which are both associated with the development of some types of cancer. By enhancing circulation, strengthening the immune system, & enhancing the body's ability to repair damaged cells, a combination of aerobic, strength training, & flexibility exercises—at least 150 minutes of moderate-intensity exercise or 75 minutes of vigorous-intensity exercise per week, as advised by the American Cancer Society—can dramatically lower the risk of cancer. Additionally, exercise encourages the release of endorphins, which can improve mood, reduce stress, & support mental health—all of which are critical for sustaining the willpower required for sustained dedication to health objectives. Regarding environmental factors, reducing exposure to carcinogens is a crucial part of any action plan for cancer prevention. Environmental toxins like air pollution, industrial chemicals, & cigarette smoke can raise the risk of developing cancer. Since tobacco use is one of the main causes of lung, throat, mouth, & several other cancers, quitting smoking & avoiding secondhand smoke are two of the best ways to lower exposure to carcinogens. Additionally, people should use natural, non-toxic cleaning products &, whenever possible, choose organic foods to reduce their exposure to environmental toxins like pesticides & household chemicals. Avoid using personal care products that contain dangerous chemicals like phthalates & parabens because they can interfere with the endocrine system & increase the risk of cancer. Reducing the risk of developing cancer requires making sure that one's home & place of employment are well-ventilated & free from excessive exposure to known carcinogens. Furthermore, preventing skin cancer—including melanoma, one of the most aggressive types of the disease—requires shielding the skin from damaging ultraviolet (UV) radiation. Effective methods for reducing the risk of skin cancer include wearing protective clothing, applying sunscreen with broad-spectrum protection, & avoiding prolonged sun exposure, particularly during peak UV hours. Additionally, it's critical to have your skin examined on a regular basis & to consult a professional if you notice any unusual moles or changes to your skin. Promoting public health regulations that restrict exposure to dangerous chemicals, air pollution, & radiation, as well as backing initiatives to lessen the environmental impact of detrimental industries, are further components of a proactive approach to environmental risk factors. A long-term cancer prevention strategy must include regular health screening & early detection procedures in addition to addressing environmental, dietary, & exercise factors. Since early-stage cancers are typically easier to treat & manage, early detection of some cancers greatly improves the likelihood of successful treatment & survival. Mammograms, colonoscopies, Pap smears, & skin examinations are examples of routine screenings that are essential for detecting possible cancers before they progress to more advanced stages. People should also be aware of the warning signs & symptoms of cancer & consult a doctor if they experience any unusual changes in their bodies, such as changes in their bowel or bladder habits, persistent pain, unexplained weight loss, or abnormal bleeding. In addition to monitoring family medical histories, routine check-ups with healthcare professionals can help detect any inherited genetic mutations that may predispose a person to cancer, allowing for early interventions or focused preventive measures. Mental wellness is another important component of long-term cancer prevention. Developing the drive & mentality required to make long-lasting lifestyle changes requires a proactive, upbeat approach to health & wellbeing. It has been demonstrated that ongoing stress impairs immunity & plays a role in the emergence of a number of illnesses, including cancer. Therefore, reducing the risk of cancer may involve implementing stress-reduction strategies into daily life. Deep breathing exercises, yoga, & meditation are examples of mindfulness practices that can help lower stress, improve emotional control, & improve mental health in general. In addition to bolstering the body's natural defences, stress management promotes a positive mental attitude that supports tenacity, self-compassion, & consistency in leading a healthy lifestyle. In addition to promoting emotional well-being, cultivating a sense of fulfilment & purpose via hobbies, social interactions, & meaningful activities can lessen the negative physical effects of stress. Additionally, maintaining a resilient mindset—which is essential for remaining dedicated to long-term health goals—is facilitated by practicing optimism, developing an attitude of gratitude, & surrounding oneself with supportive relationships. A crucial but frequently disregarded aspect of cancer prevention is social support. Creating & preserving solid, wholesome bonds with friends, family, & communities can reduce stress, promote a feeling of community, & offer emotional support. Strong social networks increase the likelihood that people will adopt healthy habits & be inspired to maintain their preventative measures. It can be simpler to stick to a prevention plan when you have an accountability partner, such as a fitness partner, support group, or medical expert, who can offer continuous encouragement & direction. Furthermore, because it can assist people in navigating uncertainty with resilience & hope, social support plays a crucial role in helping people cope with the emotional difficulties that may arise when dealing with cancer risk or the possibility of a cancer diagnosis. Last but not least, it's critical to understand that a long-term cancer prevention strategy is a continuous process that calls for constant learning, adaptation, & dedication. To make sure that preventive measures stay in line with changing individual circumstances & the most recent scientific research, it is essential to regularly reevaluate one's lifestyle, health, & risk factors. Being up to date on developments in cancer prevention, such as new screening tools, lifestyle advice, or environmental issues, enables people to modify their plans of action. Long-term success in cancer prevention requires taking an active role in one's health & well-being while staying adaptable & receptive to change. To sum up, developing a customised action plan for long-term cancer prevention requires a thorough strategy that incorporates social support, proactive health management, environmental awareness, mental wellness, & healthy lifestyle choices. It necessitates a dedication to making gradual, minor adjustments that add up to a healthier, cancer-free future. People can greatly lower their risk of developing cancer & improve their general quality of life by emphasising stress management, early detection, environmental protection, regular exercise, healthy eating, & supportive relationships. In addition to lowering the risk of cancer, a long-term cancer prevention action plan encourages a comprehensive approach to health that supports wellbeing in all facets of life. People can take charge of their health & make long-lasting changes

that promote a future of vitality, resilience, & well-being
with persistent work, education, & support.